Advance Praise for

The Wonder of Probiotics

"Dr. Taylor introduces one of the most vital and powerful aspects of health and sheds light on the many roles that pre- and probiotics play in optimal body function."

      —Jane Shellhouse, C.N., C.N.M., clinical nutritionist

"Probiotics are vital to good health, but there's a lot of mumbo jumbo and obfuscation about the choice of products on the supplement shelves. John R. Taylor, N.D., has done a great job of clearing up the confusion."

      —Lee Euler, author of *The Missing Ingredient for Good Health*

"John R. Taylor, N.D., has explored the hard evidence for probiotic supplementation for improved health. This book should be in the library of every nutritionist and physician interested in improving their patients' health."

      —Dr. Cary David Kutzke, chiropractor

The Wonder of
Probiotics

A 30-Day Plan

to Boost Energy,

Enhance Weight Loss,

Heal GI Problems,

Prevent Disease,

and Slow Aging

John R. Taylor, N.D., and Deborah Mitchell

A Lynn Sonberg Book

ST. MARTIN'S PRESS ⚏ NEW YORK

www.stmartins.com

Library of Congress Cataloging-in-Publication Data

Taylor, John R.

The wonder of probiotics : a 30-day plan to boost energy, enhance weight loss, heal GI problems, prevent disease, and slow aging / John R. Taylor and Deborah Mitchell.—1st ed.

p.   cm.

Includes bibliographical references.

ISBN-13: 978-0-312-37632-1

ISBN-10: 0-312-37632-4

1. Probiotics.   2. Intestines—Microbiology.   3. Microorganisms—Therapeutic use. 4. Dietary supplements.   I. Mitchell, Deborah R.   II. Title.

QR171.I6T39   2007

612.3'3—dc22

2007030455

10 9 8 7 6 5 4 3 2

Important Note to Readers

This book is for informational purposes only. It is not intended to take the place of medical or nutritional advice from a trained health care professional. Readers are advised to consult a physician or other qualified health professional before making any dietary changes or undertaking any new health program.

The author, proprietor, and publisher expressly disclaim responsibility for any adverse effects arising from the use or application of the information contained herein.

I dedicate this book to my wife,
Marguerite G. Taylor, N.D.,
who for nearly thirty years of marriage has been
a source of encouragement and strength to me.
And to my mother, Lois A. Taylor,
whose passing from colon cancer at age seventy-five
strengthened my resolve to educate all who will listen
about the benefits of supplementation with probiotics.
Had I known then what I know now, the story
of her life may have been written differently.

Contents

Contents

Preface:

My China Syndrome

As a naturopath and educator, a very big part of my life is involved with consulting about and recommending to clients some very tiny organisms—bacteria, in fact, and to be more specific, good bacteria known as probiotics. So when I took a recent trip to mainland China, I had a unique opportunity to test the effectiveness of probiotics in a foreign travel situation in which I would be exposed to sanitation standards different from those I was used to at home in California. Therefore, prior to my two-week jaunt around five major areas in China, I increased my normal probiotics intake as a precaution. After all, I was entering a land where swine flu, bird flu, SARS—among other infections—are known problems. I also packed several over-the-counter diarrhea medications "just in case," although, if I contracted any of the aforementioned diseases, diarrhea would likely be the least of my problems.

Our first night in Beijing was at a five-star hotel with all the amenities. As I surveyed the room before getting ready for some much-needed sleep, I saw a sign in the bathroom warning not to drink the tap water. (For the uninitiated, this warning also applies to not using the water to brush your teeth.) I knew that for the next two weeks, I would be traveling through big cities as well as some very rural areas, and U.S.-grade water would not always be easy to find. I resolved to eat and drink whatever I wanted during the entire trip—including tap water and ice made from it—and to manage my intestinal health with my arsenal of probiotics.

At that point, I was taking approximately 10 billion CFUs (I'll explain this later in the book; this is the standard form of measurement for probiotics) of twelve different good bacteria in one chewable tablet with each meal. After five to six days into the trip, I got my first "gurgle"—a little intestinal discomfort telling me that trouble could be on the horizon. One person in our tour group had already succumbed to intestinal distress and was spending the day at the hotel. I immediately doubled my probiotics dose for the next two meals, and I felt great by the next morning. I returned to my original dose of 10 billion CFUs per meal.

The sightseeing was incredible, but the schedule was very rigorous. We would leave the hotel at 7:30 AM and often not return until 10 PM, with little downtime during the day. The combination of physical stress, unusual food three times a day, questionable water supplies, and lack of sleep all contributed to a considerable stress load. I must confess that I did pass up one beverage that was offered to me: snake wine, in which rice wine is served with dead poisonous snakes coiled inside the container!

Although my tour companions took advantage of the diarrhea medications I brought with me (as well as some probiotics I offered, to get them on the road to recovery), I never had to use them myself. My intestinal health was normal for the entire trip, save the one day I increased my probiotics for two meals. Probiotics are a great travel companion!

I tell this story not to encourage you or recommend that you should recklessly drink the water against the advice of local experts whenever you travel to a foreign country. In other words, *don't try this at home, folks!* I am a trained natural health professional; I know my own system, and I was a guinea pig in my own special, controlled experiment. But what my experience *does do* is serve as an illustration of the power of probiotics, a power I know well but am constantly impressed by, as I work with clients and help them identify probiotics programs that will work best in their real-life situations.

So get prepared! Settle into a comfortable armchair and take a trip with me. You've got your ticket in your hand. Learn about probiotics and how they can transform your life for the better.

PART I

The World

of Probiotics

1

Why Everyone Needs Probiotics

There's a struggle going on in your body right now, and the participants are tireless, vigorous, and resourceful. It is a classic confrontation between two forces: good and bad. And in this case, it's between "good" or beneficial, friendly bacteria and "bad" or harmful, unfriendly bacteria. This struggle is based in your gastrointestinal tract, which covers a very large amount of territory: Stretched out, your intestinal lining covers about 300 square meters, or roughly the size of a tennis court. You are not the only one engaged in this battle. A similar one rages on in everyone regardless of age, gender, ethnicity, race, or shoe size, 24 hours a day, every day. You and your body can be the winners—or the losers—of the ongoing conflict only if you provide the friendly side with enough of the right reinforcements: Probiotics.

WHAT ARE PROBIOTICS?

Trillions of microorganisms live in your intestinal tract, or "gut," as it is commonly referred to and how we refer to it throughout this book. These beneficial flora are absolutely essential for health and well-being. If you are healthy, chances are your beneficial microorganisms are thriving as well. However, for reasons we discuss below, making sure that these friendly flora remain viable and balanced can be a challenge.

Probiotics (meaning "for life") can help you face that challenge. Probiotics are friendly, beneficial microorganisms—mainly bacteria—that work *with* the body and help maintain the delicate balance between the beneficial flora and bad bacteria that is necessary for health and well-being. When the balance tips too far in the direction of the bad bacteria, which happens frequently, a wide spectrum of symptoms and diseases can result—everything from recurring bouts of diarrhea to urinary tract infections to fatigue and muscle pain. To prevent illness as well as treat conditions associated with an imbalance between these types of bacteria, more and more health professionals and consumers are turning to probiotics, which can be found both in supplements and in a variety of foods.

Flu Busters

I'm going to take a moment here to share a personal story about the power of probiotics because it's a tale with which many people can identify. How many times in your life have you been floored by the flu? You know the symptoms: nausea, vomiting, diarrhea, aches, and generally feeling lousy. Like the zit that erupts on your face the day you have an important date or need to give a big presentation, the flu often appears at very inconvenient times. So, when I woke up on the morning of the big annual chili cookoff competition that my family sponsors every year at our house and I was overwhelmed by nausea, vomiting, diarrhea, and fever, I knew I was in trouble. I had approximately eight hours to get better, before hordes of people would appear on my doorstep carrying steaming crockpots full of spicy, hot chili.

Fortunately, I knew what I had to do: I immediately took 2.5 billion CFUs (colony-forming units—the number of viable cells in a dose) of five species of probiotics and went to bed. Then every two hours for the next eight hours, I took 2.5 billion CFUs of probiotics and continued to rest. By the time the first chili competitors rang my doorbell at 5 PM, I was free of symptoms: no more nausea, vomiting, diarrhea, or fever. However, I thought better of diving headfirst into the waiting bowls of chili, so when the competition heated up a few hours later, I ate conservatively, just sampling many different chilis. Throughout that night and the next day, I continued to take about 2.5 billion CFUs of probiotics every six to eight hours. Within seven to eight hours of experiencing my first flu symptoms, I was not only symptom-free, but felt like my old self.

This is just one example of the power of probiotics. Since that chili adventure, I have used this probiotic treatment approach several more times, and it has worked every time. Without getting into a detailed discussion of how and why probiotics work—which we do in chapter 2 and in part two of this book—here we want to say that, when you provide probiotics to your gut—in food and/or supplements—your goal is to tilt the balance of bacteria highly in favor of the good guys, so they can effectively inhibit the growth and development of unfriendly bacterial strains and prevent other pathogens from staking a claim in the body.

Balancing Bacteria

Why is this balance so hard to maintain? A quick look at modern society and lifestyles provides the answer. Literally dozens of factors make it difficult to maintain the critical balance between beneficial and harmful bacteria. Poor food choices, use of antibiotics and other drugs, emotional stress, lack of sleep, environmental influences—all of these factors and more jeopardize the balance in the intestinal flora, resulting in a reduction of beneficial bacteria and opening the door for bad bacteria and other disease-causing substances (pathogens) to take over and cause infection, illness, and disease. Bad bacteria are also very opportunistic, prime examples of the old adage, "give an inch, take a mile." If the environment in your gut is even mildly favorable to bad bacteria, they will grow and proliferate with a vengeance.

The challenge, then, is to provide your body with plenty of friendly bacteria to thwart the actions of the bad bacteria and other pathogens, and to restore a healthy balance in your gut.

MORE ABOUT THE GUT

By the time you finish this book—or perhaps even this chapter—you should have a newfound appreciation for your gut and all the complex and health-maintaining activities that go on there. We hope to help you understand that what happens in your gut significantly impacts every cell, tissue, and organ system in your body.

The Glorious Gut

The intestinal tract is a remarkable organ that is coated with both friendly and unfriendly microorganisms which, together with the actual cell lining of the gut, serve both as a protective barrier and a filtering and distribution point. When the gut is healthy, it successfully filters out and eliminates damaging substances such as unfriendly bacteria, toxins, chemicals, and other waste products, and prevents them from being absorbed and carried throughout the body. At the same time, the gut absorbs and helps distribute essential ingredients, such as nutrients from food and water, and sends them to the cells in the body that need them.

Thus, the gut has a great deal of control over what happens throughout your body, just like the brain in your head controls your bodily functions. This association between gut and brain is more than coincidence, it's a physical reality.

The Brain-Gut Axis

In fact, scientists have found that a network of chemical and electrical signals continuously pass between the central nervous system (brain) and the gastrointestinal system. They call this exchange pathway the *brain-gut axis,* and some experts refer to the gut as the *second brain.* This intimate relationship between your cerebral brain and your gut brain is one reason why what happens in your gut has such an effect on the rest of the body.

The truth is, most people are pretty hard on their second brain. For example, think about your diet. Do you consume processed foods, fried foods, sugar, alcohol? How about foods that contain pesticides, antibiotics, hormones, steroids, artificial colors, preservatives, and flavorings? These dietary assaults on your gut, and many other factors (discussed below), can cause the bacterial flora in your gut to go out of balance.

Once the beneficial flora decline in number, damaging substances gain the upper hand and your health suffers: Your gut becomes damaged and inflamed, toxins get into your bloodstream and cause distressing symptoms, nutritional deficiencies occur, and a host of other health conditions can result.

That's why the basis of any health or healing plan must focus lots of attention on your gut. Exactly what makes the gut so important?

The Gut at Work

The intestinal tract is the distribution point for nutrients throughout your body. If your distribution center isn't working properly, the nutrients don't get sent to their required destinations. What would happen if the sorting system at your local post office went on the blink, half the employees didn't show up for work, and the trucks broke down? The mail would enter the post office, but it couldn't be sorted or distributed, and you wouldn't get your mail. Your gut works in a similar way: You can put food and nutrients into your body, but if your gut isn't healthy enough to support and handle them, they will not get processed and distributed throughout your body.

The colon is the main channel for bad bacteria, medication residues, parasites, and other toxins and waste to leave the body. It is essential that these materials leave the body regularly and as completely as possible. Yet, poor dietary habits and lifestyle practices cause many people to suffer from incomplete elimination and to retain fecal matter much longer—even years—and in great quantities in their intestinal tract. Not only does old fecal matter offer a perfect environment in which bad bacteria can breed and grow, it also causes the walls of the colon to expand and press on other organs in the abdominal cavity, ultimately resulting in conditions such as polyps, colon cancer, diverticulosis, and Crohn's disease.

Hardened fecal matter on the walls of the colon also make it very difficult for you to absorb any nutrients from your food. This can result in nutritional deficiencies. In fact, the whole relationship between health, probiotics, incomplete elimination, and residual fecal matter is so important that we address it in more detail in chapter 4, where you can learn how to cultivate healthy bowel habits that will enhance your overall health and vitality.

If you consume probiotics every day, as food and/or supplements, you can help maintain the proper balance of bacterial flora in the gut and thus enjoy better health and vitality. We will explore the unique relationship between beneficial bacteria and health in each of the chapters in part two, where we talk about how probiotics can help specific symptoms and medical conditions.

HOW DO YOU KNOW IF YOU NEED PROBIOTICS?

I like to think about good and bad bacteria and the gut in terms of mosquitoes and swamps. If you were to stand in a swamp (i.e., a gut that is swarming with bad bacteria), you could swat at the great hordes of swarming mosquitoes all day with a fly swatter and you would never kill an appreciable number, as long as the bugs have the swamp in which to reproduce and grow. If you were to drain the swamp, you would remove the mosquitoes' resource for life, and they would die. Similarly, if you were to scoop up a bottle full of mosquitoes and release them in a pristine, dry environment in which there were no bodies of water where the mosquitoes could breed and reproduce, they would die.

Thus you have a choice: Your gut can be a nasty swamp and a breeding ground for unfriendly bacteria and other pathogens, which places you at constant risk of an extensive range of illnesses and diseases; or you can drain the swamp—chase out all those nasty bacteria—and provide a friendly, pristine environment that supports and nurtures beneficial bacteria, good health, and vitality.

The Impact of Lifestyle

One important reason why you need to keep replenishing your beneficial bacteria levels is that outside forces—things you do every day—are constantly causing their numbers to be reduced. Decades of research by experts around the world, including the groundbreaking work of Dr. Khem Shahani, arguably the foremost authority on probiotics, have shown that an imbalance between friendly and unfriendly bacteria in the gut can be caused or worsened by unwise lifestyle choices, including a poor diet, and environmental factors.

Unfortunately, these lifestyle choices and environmental factors have become status quo for many people. I can't tell you how many people have come to me complaining of fatigue, gastrointestinal problems, recurring infections, and other health issues, and when I question them about their lifestyle habits I see that they are "living their problem": They're eating fast food, lots of sugar and sugary foods, and foods that contain hormones, antibiotics, steroids, artificial colors and preservatives, and other contaminants. They don't get enough sleep and they don't manage their stress well. Many women tell me they are taking birth control pills and that they have a history of taking antibiotics, often for urinary tract or yeast infections. And without fail, everyone is exposed to environmental stressors, including secondhand smoke, greenhouse gases, chlorinated and/or fluoridated water, and household and workplace chemicals. The good news is that many of the items I've just listed involve choices, which means you have the power to change them. People can do much to make positive changes in their lives while adding probiotics to the picture.

While keeping the lifestyle choices and environmental factors in mind, look at the following statements about health and well-being. How many are true about you?

- Frequent tension headache and/or migraine are a problem for me.
- It's common for me to wake up tired and to feel tired all day long.
- I experience bouts of constipation and/or diarrhea.

- I often experience bloating and/or gas.
- I have had candida (yeast) infections.
- I occasionally or frequently get urinary tract infections.
- My skin is often itchy, and/or I have psoriasis, eczema, acne, or rash.
- I experience frequent colds and/or flu.
- I often get anxious and/or depressed.
- I experience some memory problems.
- I have asthma and/or nasal allergies.
- No matter how hard I try, I have trouble losing weight.
- My cholesterol is high.
- I frequently get cold sores.
- I'm experiencing symptoms of perimenopause, menopause, or PMS.
- I have chronic bad breath.

The vast majority of people say yes to three or more of these statements, and many find that more than half of the statements are true for them. This is not unusual. Studies show that these complaints, as well as many diseases and other medical conditions, are associated with an imbalance (or "dysbiosis") between good and bad bacteria in the gut. These conditions include bowel disorders (e.g., irritable bowel syndrome, Crohn's disease, colitis, inflammatory bowel disease), migraine, chronic fatigue syndrome, cancer, chronic inflammation, psoriasis, eczema, fibromyalgia, acne, and autoimmune disorders.

Probiotics and Antibiotics

Most people who are familiar with or who have heard about probiotics associate them with antibiotics, and in fact this is often the first way people are introduced to probiotics. This is a fortunate introduction, and one I want to explain here, because the relationship between antibiotics and probiotics is a good illustration of how the use of beneficial bacteria can enhance your health and well-being.

If you consider these two words—*pro*biotics and *anti*biotics—you can readily see that they have something in common. Antibiotics are drugs that are prescribed to destroy life—the life of disease-causing bacteria in the body—and in many cases these drugs do this quite well and save many lives and relieve much suffering in the process. Probiotics promote or give life, and they do a very admirable job, as you will learn throughout this book. Yet, unlike probiotics, antibiotics also have a sinister side: Not only do they destroy bad bacteria, but they destroy beneficial bacteria as well. And even though this is a well-known medical fact, antibiotics continue to be abused and misused on a large scale.

For example, despite the fact that antibiotics are *not* effective against viruses such as the common cold and flu, these drugs are still being prescribed for viral conditions, resulting in widespread antibiotic resistance and thus placing people's health in jeopardy. One recommendation in such cases, as my experience with the flu and my chili adventure illustrates, is to avoid antibiotics and instead take probiotics.

When antibiotics are medically indicated for a bacterial infection such as bacterial pneumonia or a wound infection, then it is strongly recommended that people take a probiotic supplement before, during, and/or after a course of antibiotics to help restore the healthy bacteria in their gut. We'll talk more about the use of antibiotics and probiotics in chapter 8. For now, however, we just want to let you know that although it is very important to take probiotics while you are also using antibiotics, to help offset the damage caused by the drugs, it is by no means the *only* way you can harness the power of these beneficial microorganisms in your life.

WHAT CAN PROBIOTICS DO FOR YOU?

The organisms in probiotics may be microscopic, but they can take on some very big roles. Some people consider them to be like an insurance policy: Use of probiotics allows them to ward off potential infections and other health problems and provides them with a more healthy foundation.

"I feel like I have a health-care policy in force, just in case something does happen," explains Vivian, a forty-nine-year-old interior designer, "plus, using probiotics regularly offers me peace of mind."

Millions of people are like Vivian, and you may be among them: You don't have any pressing health issues or symptoms—perhaps you experience an occasional headache or cold, infrequent bouts of constipation or diarrhea, but nothing serious—but your diet could be much better. You're often under pressure at work and like everyone else, you can't escape the greenhouse gases in the air you breathe. For you, a simple plan to include probiotics in your diet and/or with supplements is a wise way to safeguard your health.

Or you may be among the growing number of parents who are turning to probiotics and their helpers as a way to protect, enhance, and improve the health and well-being of their infants and children. This is an area that I find especially rewarding and a topic I want to discuss right up front because it is so important to so many people.

Probiotics and Children

People often wonder if probiotics are recommended for infants and children, and the answer is a resounding *Yes!* In fact, in chapters 5 and 6 especially, which explore gastrointestinal problems and allergies and asthma respectively, you'll learn just how critical probiotics can be in the treatment and prevention of life-threatening diarrhea and respiratory conditions, including asthma, that affect a growing number of our children.

I talk to a great number of mothers of infants who contact me because their children are colicky or are having continuous bouts of green diarrhea. I explain to them that the intestinal tract of infants cannot mature without an adequate population of beneficial bacteria. Every child is born with a clean "slate": a sterile intestinal tract. Microorganisms begin to move in and multiply as soon as the infant is born. In fact, infants tend to swallow some vaginal fluid at delivery, and because vaginal bacteria and intestinal bacteria are similar, an infant's bacterial flora will generally be similar to that of his or her mother. Thus, if the mother's intestinal flora is unbalanced, that imbalance is passed along to the infant as well. Infants who are delivered via cesarean section are not exposed to the mother's vaginal fluids and often acquire bacterial flora that is present in the delivery room or hospital environment.

The main source of bacteria that eventually colonize the gut, however, is food. Infants who are breast-fed enjoy the many benefits of colostrum (the fluid that is secreted from the mother's breast before the breast milk appears) and breast milk. These wonder foods of nature contain antibodies, antiviral substances, vitamins, prebiotics (which we talk about in detail in chapter 3), and other essential ingredients that help prepare the infant's gut and immune system for life's challenges. *Bifidobacteria* species are the predominant good bacteria in breast-fed infants, and they typically multiply rapidly and appear in the feces of infants within a few days of birth. In infants who are given formula, other bacteria, including clostridia, bacteroides, streptococci, as well as *Bifidobacteria* appear. The fewer number of *Bifidobacteria* species in formula-fed infants is one of the main reasons why these children tend to experience significantly more episodes of diarrhea, ear infections, and other common health problems than do breast-fed infants.

Attaining and maintaining a healthy balance of friendly and unfriendly bacteria in the gut is critically important in infants and children. For example, diarrhea can be life-threatening to an infant or very young child, and so, restoring a healthy balance of beneficial bacteria is a crucial part of the treatment and recovery process. Researchers have also found that some allergies originate in childhood among children who have a deficiency of friendly bacteria, which means they are more likely to have an underdeveloped gastrointestinal tract and a less than robust immune system as adults.

Probiotics for All

You may be one of tens of millions of Americans who has an annoying, chronic, or significant health challenge that can be relieved, managed, or eliminated through use of probiotics. Are you among the nearly 45 million Americans who, according to the International Foundation for Functional Gastrointestinal Disorders, suffers with irritable bowel syndrome? Or are you one of the 75 percent of adult women who will suffer with at least one, and often more, episodes of vaginal candidiasis? Is your child among the 9 million U.S. youngsters under age eighteen who has been diagnosed with asthma? Are you or other family members having trouble losing weight and keeping it off?

Probiotics are especially important for those who can't vocalize a "yes" to any of these statements—infants and very young children— who often fall victim to diarrhea and other gastrointestinal problems, as we mentioned above. And for those who share their homes with four-legged companions, probiotics can be beneficial for many canine and feline ailments as well. (Yes, we talk about probiotics for pets in chapter 12.)

Probiotics can play a crucial role in all of the situations mentioned here, and more. If it sounds like probiotics are some kind of "miracle" substance that's too good to be true, let me assure you that that is not the case.

Beneficial bacteria occur naturally in the body, but they need constant support and restoration. Providing the body with an adequate and reliable supply of good bacteria in the form of probiotics is not magic, it is wise behavior, scientifically proven to work to provide optimum health. And that's the kind of behavior we encourage in this book.

Our hope is that you will embrace the use of probiotics not only for yourself, but for your entire family, including your children. In fact, helping to ensure your children have a healthy balance of beneficial bacteria in their gut now is one of the best and easiest ways to arm them against illness and disease, both now and in their future years.

HOW TO USE THIS BOOK

This book is divided into two parts. Part one consists of three chapters, including this one, in which we introduce you to the world of probiotics and their health-balancing, restorative powers. Many people have heard the word "probiotics," but have little or no idea what they are, how they work, or, more important, the many ways they can improve their health and restore a higher quality of life. Therefore, these few chapters can help you understand and appreciate the power of these microorganisms, the many different types of beneficial bacteria that are available in both supplement form and in foods, how easy it is to incorporate them into your lifestyle, and how you can enhance their performance when they are combined with selected "little helpers," all natural prebiotics and enzymes.

Part two presents more than a dozen different easy-to-follow probiotic programs. Each one addresses a different health challenge that you can remedy through the use of probiotic supplements and/or selected foods and probiotic helpers. Each chapter begins with an overview of the medical condition(s) or health problem(s), including a checklist, so you can better identify your signs and symptoms. The one exception to this is chapter 4, which presents a probiotic program that is for anyone who doesn't have a specific ailment but who wants to enhance their overall health, experience more energy, and enjoy a better quality of life. This basic, core probiotic program is virtually for everyone and, like all the other programs in part two it is easy to follow.

In 1996, the World Health Report stated that "too few new drugs are being developed to replace those that have lost their effectiveness. In the race for supremacy, microbes are sprinting ahead." Although drugs do have their place in the fight against microbes and in dealing with the symptoms of disease, in many cases what we need are not more drugs, but making sure that people are getting enough probiotics in their lives, whether through their food or supplements or both. This book shows you how to make probiotics work for you.

2

Probiotics: An Inside Look

at How They Work

Right now, your intestinal tract is harboring three to four pounds of microorganisms (that translates into about 25 trillion microorganisms per pound, give or take a few trillion), a population comprised of four to five hundred different species of bacteria. Should you be alarmed by the presence of these tiny inhabitants in your body? No—in fact, they make up three to four pounds that you *don't* want to lose, because they play a key role in your overall health.

A few hundred different species may sound like a mere drop in the bucket (or in your gut) when compared with trillions of microorganisms, but an even smaller proportion—thirty to forty different species—make up 99 percent of the total different species of bacteria that reside there. Among all these species of bacteria are both friendly and unfriendly varieties. Experts say that, ideally, you want the scale to tip largely in favor of the beneficial bacteria—say, about 85 percent friendly versus 15 percent unfriendly. That's what it takes to help hold the vigorous unfriendly bacteria at bay. One of the primary purposes of this book is to tell you how to do that easily.

Unfortunately, many people have a gut whose bacterial flora is far from the 85/15 goal, and they have the signs, symptoms, and health problems to show for it. The good news is that it isn't difficult to swing the balance back in favor of beneficial bacteria in your gut, and thus dramatically improve your health.

Here are just a few of the many jobs beneficial bacteria perform:

- aid in digestion
- assist in the absorption of nutrients
- help prevent skin problems
- fight yeast and fungal infections, including candida
- stimulate function of the immune system
- keep pathogens (disease-causing organisms) in check
- prevent and control diarrhea
- enhance calcium metabolism, which helps prevent osteoporosis
- help maintain a balance of pH
- help produce vitamin K and B vitamins
- help regulate activity of the bowel
- help decrease the number of carcinogenic components in the intestinal tract
- inhibit the formation of tumors
- assist in liver function and detoxification
- reduce the accumulation of cholesterol and plaque in the arteries

You are probably saying to yourself, "Okay, you've told me that beneficial bacteria can do a lot of wonderful things for my health, so now tell me exactly how I can cash in on these health benefits!" We'll get to that, I promise. But first I strongly encourage you to read this chapter and the one that follows. I guarantee you will learn things about beneficial bacteria and probiotics that will help you more fully understand

and appreciate the full range of their capabilities and, what is more important, how to use them and their helpers to your best advantage. Wouldn't you like to know more about the billions of bacteria you are going to welcome into your gut? Then read on and discover the different types of probiotics, the many different symptoms and diseases they can prevent and treat, the intricate relationship they have with other health-enhancing substances, and the improvements they can bring to your life.

EXPLAINING PROBIOTICS

For the sake of clarity, it's worth pointing out the difference between beneficial microorganisms (also referred to as beneficial bacteria or beneficial flora) and probiotics. Beneficial microorganisms exist naturally in the body: they reproduce, perform their many functions, and die. Probiotics are also beneficial microorganisms, but they are *introduced into* the body via supplements and/or foods that contain beneficial organisms, in an effort to replenish declining levels of these friendly organisms.

Probiotics are nothing new: Even though people in ancient times didn't call these organisms probiotics, they recognized that something good happened when they consumed soured (fermented) milk and cultured dairy products. Such foods, including yogurt, kefir, and *dahi* (a type of yogurt) are mentioned in the sacred books of Hinduism and in the Bible and are noted for their healing qualities. In fact, fermented milk products have been a major part of the human diet for people throughout Africa, Asia, and Eastern Europe for millennia. Fermentation is one of the oldest methods for preserving food, and even today many cultures throughout Asia, Africa, and Eastern Europe use fermented foods as part of their daily diet. Not coincidentally, the people in these cultures enjoy a healthy balance of beneficial bacteria in their gastrointestinal tract. (See box, "What Is Fermentation?")

What Is Fermentation?

Fermentation is a complex process; but in simple terms, it refers to the use of microorganisms—enzymes, bacteria, molds, and/or yeasts—on or in food to change the characteristics of the food. These microorganisms convert nutrients, such as sugars, mainly into lactic acid, acetic acid, and ethanol, as well as some other substances. *Lactobacillus, Bifidobacterium,* and *Streptococcus,* for example, are bacteria that convert nutrients into lactic acid, which is why they are referred to as lactic acid bacteria (see "Meet the Probiotics").

Common fermented foods include yogurt, pickles, sauerkraut, and sourdough breads, while many others may be less familiar or even strange. However, fermented foods are very popular in many cultures around the world and are consumed daily. The fact that fermentation involves allowing foods to "sit" for many hours at or near room temperature causes some people to think that these foods cannot be safe and that they are breeding grounds for bad bacteria. In fact, fermented foods are extremely safe and are commonly consumed in developing countries where poor sanitary conditions exist. That's because the beneficial and edible microorganisms grown on these foods virtually eliminate the risk of contamination with disease-causing organisms such as *Salmonella* and *Clostridium*. The presence of lactic acid is responsible not only for the sour taste (sour pickles, sauerkraut), but also for the safety of the food. You can learn more about fermented foods and how to include them in your daily diet in chapter 12.

The official definition of probiotics, according to the Food and Agriculture Organization of the United Nations (FAO), is "live microorganisms administered in adequate amounts, which confer a beneficial health effect on the host." Therefore, throughout this book we make the distinction between these two similar groups whenever possible, although there are some cases in which use of either word or phrase is appropriate, including the case here.

Five Criteria for Probiotics

Not just any microorganism has what it takes to be a probiotic. To qualify as a beneficial microorganism and thus earn the title of "probiotic," the following criteria must be met:

1. It must be resistant to bile and acids.
2. It must be able to attach itself successfully to the gastrointestinal tract.
3. It must be able to remain metabolically active once it reaches the gastrointestinal tract.
4. It must be able to damage, destroy, or otherwise render harmless disease-causing (pathogenic) bacteria.
5. It must balance pH levels in the colon.

Now that you know what it takes to be a probiotic, you should know that, of the hundreds of different bacteria experts have identified thus far, only a few dozen can be counted among the beneficial bacteria you want to welcome into your gut, and only some of them can be stabilized properly so they can be delivered to you in an effective form in either a supplement or food, such as yogurt or acidophilus milk.

A Little Bit of History

In the late nineteenth century, microbiologists discovered that the microorganisms in the gastrointestinal tracts of healthy people differed from those in people who were ill, and they dubbed the good organisms "probiotics." Soon thereafter, a Russian biologist and Nobel Prize winner, Dr. Elie Metchnikoff, was conducting research among long-lived Bulgarians and proposed that their longevity was related to their ingestion of fermented milk products. He was quite confident that these foods—especially yogurt in the case of the Bulgarians—helped maintain the good balance of microorganisms in the gastrointestinal tract. To memorialize his finding, Dr. Metchnikoff named the main yogurt-culturing bacteria *Lactobacillus bulgaricus*.

Dr. Metchnikoff presented many of his findings in his 1907 book, *The Prolongation of Life,* in which he noted that people who ate yogurt that contained live bacteria such as *Lactobacillus bulgaricus* and *Streptococcus thermophilus* experienced better gastrointestinal and overall health, and also enjoyed increased longevity. Subsequently, both of these probiotic bacteria became the standard starter strains for the production of yogurt around the world.

PROBIOTICS

Daphne was confused. "My friend Janet told me that she was taking probiotic supplements because she had had a yeast infection, and the supplements cleared it up. Then she said she was still taking the supplements because they were like insurance against getting the infection again. Since I had had a yeast infection recently as well, I thought I'd get some probiotics, too. But when I went to my health food store and asked for probiotics, they asked me which ones I wanted. Which ones? I didn't know there was more than one kind!"

Not only are there several different varieties of beneficial bacteria, but each one has one or more different health benefits that it offers, or jobs that it can perform. Despite their individual differences, however, all the different beneficial bacteria that we discuss here can be placed in a general category called "lactic acid bacteria." (Note: The probiotic yeast *Saccharomyces boulardii* does not fall into this category.) This means that the bacteria have the ability to transform sugar into lactic acid, a substance that can destroy unfriendly, disease-causing bacteria, much like antibiotics do, but without the side effects that accompany antibiotics. Lactic acid is also the substance that is necessary for the production of fermented foods such as yogurt, some cheeses, and sauerkraut. (See: "What Is Fermentation?")

All probiotics are also anaerobic organisms. That means they do not require oxygen to survive, and they can thrive in a dark, warm environment, like your gut. (Some probiotics can live both with or without oxygen.) The ability of probiotics to thrive without oxygen is an important point to remember, and we will discuss it later in this book.

All probiotics are categorized according to genus and species, and often strain names (a subcategory of species) as well. The probiotic most people recognize by name is acidophilus, which officially is known as *Lactobacillus acidophilus,* or *L. acidophilus* for short, although there are various strains of this bacteria, as you will learn below. Some strains have been studied extensively, including the *L. acidophilus* DDS-1, which was the focus of study by Dr. Shahani; and *Lactobacillus GG,* the beneficial bacteria thoroughly investigated by two Boston scientists. Both of these strains, as well as other commonly used probiotics, are discussed here.

Lactobacillus sp.

The lactobacilli are among the most common beneficial bacteria that live in the gut. They also populate the vagina, which is important to remember once we talk about probiotics and infections of the reproductive tract (chapter 7). Thus far, more than fifty species of *Lactobacillus* have been identified. Some of those used as probiotics include the following (if you look at the label on yogurt that contains live cultures, you may see one or more of these probiotics listed): *L. acidophilus* strains DDS-1, BG2FO4, INT-9, NCFB 1748, NCFM, and SBT-2062; *L. brevis; L. bulgaricus; L. casei* and *L. casei Shirota; L. cellobiosus; L. crispatus; L. delbrueckii* subspecies *delbrueckii* and *L. delbrueckii* subspecies *bulgaricus* type 2038; *L. fermentum; L. GG (L. rhamnosus* or *L. casei* subspecies *rhamnosus); L. plantarum,* and *L. salivarus.*

The *Lactobacillus* species perform many beneficial functions. For example, they preserve vitamins and antioxidants in the body, remove toxic food elements, prevent food decay, and block damage caused by unfriendly bacteria (e.g., *S. aureus, Enterococci,* and *Enterobacteriaceae)* found in fermented foods.

Here is a closer look at some of the more effective *Lactobacillus* species.

- *Lactobacillus acidophilus.* This species of beneficial bacteria can produce natural antibiotics (e.g., acidolin, lactocidin, acidophilin), including antiviral compounds. It is also capable of inhibiting the growth of some very common pathogens, including *Salmonella, Shigella, Enterococcus faecalis,* and *E. coli,* which can cause, among other things, diarrhea, abdominal cramps, vomiting, inflammation of the gastrointestinal tract, and infections of the genital tract. *Lactobacillus acidophilus* is found naturally in both the large and small intestine, as well as in the mouth and vagina.

- *L. acidophilus* DDS-1. This special *Lactobacillus* strain has been the subject of extensive research for decades at the University of Nebraska, originally under the careful eye of Dr. Khem Shahani. Beginning in 1959, Dr. Shahani conducted research on finding and developing the best strains of beneficial bacteria, and *L. acidophilus* DDS-1 emerged as "the friendliest flora" of them all. This strain is unique among probiotics because it is more resistant to heat and to the severe environment in the intestinal tract, which makes it better able to destroy and prevent the colonization and reproduction of unfriendly bacteria, and maintain a healthy balance in the gut. One very important property of this strain is its ability to resist antibiotics, which means you can take this probiotic even while you are taking an antibiotic, and thus help prevent an imbalance of bacterial flora in your gut caused by the medication.
- *Lactobacillus bulgaricus.* In the United States, this species must be used along with *Streptococcus thermophilus* in the production of yogurt. It has also demonstrated antitumor properties in several studies.
- *Lactobacillus ramnosus GG.* *Lactobacillus* GG (so named after the two scientists, Sherwood Gorbach and Barry Goldin, who first isolated it) is a strain of lactobacilli that has many beneficial properties, including a superior ability to prevent and treat gastrointestinal disorders, especially diarrhea in both children and adults. It is also very effective in the prevention and treatment of viral and bacterial infections, and as an immune system enhancer. Some of the features that make *Lactobacillus* GG so important are its ability to resist acid and bile and to survive the trip from the stomach to the intestinal tract, all of which make it a good choice to include in yogurt cultures and other fermented foods. *Lactobacillus* GG is so respected in Japan that the Japanese have used it

in the first and only food that has been developed solely as a probiotic.

- *Lactobacillus plantarium.* Research shows that this species works along with *L. acidophilus* to destroy pathogens. It also possesses the unusual ability to produce *L. lysine*, a beneficial amino acid, and to preserve critical nutrients, vitamins, and antioxidants.

- *Lactobacillus reuteri.* This species is more effective as an antibiotic than its cousin, *L. acidophilus.* Recent studies in Sweden also show that this probiotic appears to protect infants and young children against the development of allergies and other allergy respiratory diseases.

- *Lactobacillus salivarius.* Most intestinal disorders respond very well to this probiotic. This species is also used to strengthen the immune system.

- *Lactobacillus casei.* The *casei* strains of the *Lactobacillus* genus are found naturally in fermented vegetables, milk, and meat, and reside in the gut, human mouth, and environment. They are smaller in size than some of the other *Lactobacillus* species and complement the growth of *L. acidophilus. L. casei*, and improve digestion and reduce lactose intolerance and constipation. And if you enjoy beans and chili, then this species of *Lactobacillus* will be especially interesting for you: Researchers in Venezuela have discovered that when they fermented beans with *L. casei*, they reduced the flatulence-causing ingredient by 88 percent and increased insoluble fiber by 97 percent.

Bifidobacteria sp.

Approximately 90 percent of the beneficial bacteria in a healthy colon are *Bifidobacteria* species. These friendly anaerobic lactic acid bacteria take up residence in the colon within days of birth, especially in infants who are breast-fed, and remain a critical factor in gastrointestinal, immune, and overall health throughout a lifetime.

Approximately thirty species of *Bifidobacteria* have been identified and isolated, and those used as probiotics include *B. adolescentis, B. bifidum, B. animalis, B. thermophilum, B. breve* strains Yakult and RO7O; *B. longum* strains RO23, SBT-2928, and BB536; *B. bifidum RO71; B. infantis* strain RO33; and *B. lactis* strain Bb12.

Along with lactic acid, *Bifidobacteria* also produce acetic acid, and together these acids reduce the pH in the intestinal tract, which in turn inhibits the growth of potentially disease-causing organisms. *Bifidobacteria* are more effective than *Lactobacillus* when it comes to fighting and destroying pathogens, because the former produces more acetic acid, and the acid is better utilized by the intestinal tract. Many of the *Bifidobacteria* species also synthesize and excrete water-soluble vitamins (primarily the B vitamin family) and help metabolize carbohydrates.

- *Bifidobacteria bifidum.* This species is especially effective in suppressing the activity of harmful bacteria and other pathogens. It is the main bacterial component in the human large intestine, but is also found in the small intestine and mouth. *B. bifidum* produces B vitamins.
- *Bifidobacteria lactis.* Among the benefits of this species are its ability to lower the body's pH and to inhibit the growth of unfriendly bacteria. One reason it excels at destroying pathogens is that it produces hydrogen peroxide, which is an antibacterial agent.
- *Bifidobacteria longum.* Prevention of gastrointestinal problems is the main benefit of this probiotic, which it does by crowding out unfriendly bacteria in the gut.

Lactococci

Lactococci are lactic acid bacteria that are often used to ferment milk products, including cheese. These beneficial bacteria are not naturally present in the gut, although some studies have found them there. What's important is that these bacteria have shown that they can reduce cholesterol levels (see chapter 9). They also have the ability to inhibit the growth of unfriendly bacteria. You may find some of these beneficial bacteria in various probiotic products: *L. lactis, L. lactis* subspecies *cremoris,* subspecies *lactis* NCDO 712, subspecies *lactis* NIAI 527, and subspecies NIAI 1061, among others.

Saccharomyces boulardii

Saccharomyces boulardii is the only yeast probiotic that has been identified thus far. It is closely related to brewer's yeast, but it is not at all related to the yeast *Candida,* which causes candidiasis. When *Saccharomyces boulardii* is taken as a supplement, it quickly establishes itself in the gut and helps eliminate harmful yeast species. It also has the ability to produce lactic acid and some B vitamins. Among the conditions most effectively treated with *S. boulardii* are diarrhea associated with the use of antibiotics and maintenance treatment for Crohn's disease (see chapter 8).

Streptococcus thermophilus

This lactic acid bacteria is found in milk and milk products, and is usually used along with *L. bulgaricus* to make yogurt and mozzarella cheese. *Streptococcus thermophilus* is very effective in the prevention of lactose intolerance, as this species produces large quantities of the enzyme lactase. Both *S. thermophilus* and another strain, *S. salivarus* subspecies *thermophilus* type 1131, are used as probiotics.

THE WONDER OF PROBIOTICS

Enterococcus faecium

Enterococci are normally found in the intestinal tract of both humans and animals. *Enterococcus faecium* is a strain that colonizes the gut only temporarily. The strain that is most often used as a probiotic to prevent and treat diarrhea is *E. faecium* SF68. *E. faecium* is very hardy; unlike most other probiotics, it is able to withstand the high acidic levels and temperatures found in the stomach, and in fact helps other beneficial bacteria to become established in the gut. It is also very resistant to many different antibiotics.

Enterococcus faecium also appears to be helpful in lowering cholesterol levels. In one recent study, for example, the M-74 strain of these beneficial bacteria decreased serum cholesterol levels by 12 percent in a group of men and women volunteers. For now, however, *E. faecium* is most often used for people who have diarrhea, especially those with diarrhea associated with rotavirus. (See chapter 5 for a more detailed discussion about diarrhea and probiotics.)

Fighting the Bad Guys

Now that you've met the good guys, it's time to meet some of the bad bacteria. Unfriendly bacteria are responsible for a wide variety of ailments and diseases, and so it's advantageous to put them out of commission. In the intestinal tract, the unfriendly bacteria can cause illness and disease when the population of beneficial bacteria is insufficient to fight them off. The most common harmful bacteria in the gut include the following:

- *Clostridium.* Some of the more common species in this genus include *C. botulinum* (causes food poisoning and is one of the most deadly toxins in existence), *C. difficile* (diarrhea), *C. perfringens* (infection, diarrhea), and *C. tetani* (tetanus).
- *Escherichia* (some strains). Some strains of the *E. coli* species are

the number-one cause of urinary tract infections. They are also responsible for diarrhea, meningitis, pneumonia, and many other conditions. On the positive side, some *E. coli* strains help produce vitamin K in the large intestine.

- Coliform. Coliform bacteria are commonly found in the environment and usually cause little or no health problems. However, when they are found in drinking water, this is often an indication that human or animal waste has contaminated the water supply. Crops irrigated with contaminated water, as was the case in the fall of 2006, when lettuce grown in California's Salinas Valley was recalled because *E. coli*–contaminated water had been used in irrigation. One particular strain of *E. coli,* strain O157:H7, has been responsible for many deaths and hundreds of thousands of cases of food poisoning in the United States and elsewhere. Symptoms of exposure to coliform bacteria include cramps, bloody stools, diarrhea, headache, nausea, and vomiting, and in severe cases, paralysis, kidney failure, respiratory failure, and death.

- *Staphylococcus.* Among the many species, *S. aureus* is associated with soft tissue infection and food poisoning. *S. epidermis* causes skin infections.

- *Pseudomonas.* This genus is important because it is very resistant to most antibiotics, is often found in hospitals and clinics, and is a major cause of hospital-acquired infections. It most often affects immunocompromised individuals, especially hospitalized or nursing home patients.

Another genus, *Bacteroides,* makes up the majority of microorganisms in the digestive tract. However, the species associated with this genus rarely cause any type of infection or illness. About 50 percent of fecal matter is composed of *Bacteroides fragilis* cells.

Unfriendly bacteria also produce toxic substances that place the body in a state of constant stress. When you significantly reduce the production of these toxins, you can help your body heal. Probiotics stimulate the immune system and help it suppress the growth of further disease-causing bacteria. This is especially important once you learn how probiotics are effective in fighting and preventing the return of conditions that often recur, such as urinary tract infections, candida, and other yeast infections.

Where Have All the Beneficial Bacteria Gone?

A number of probiotics that belong to the genus *Lactobacilli*, which we explain in detail in this chapter, unfortunately are in short supply among the general population in the United States and among other people living in industrialized countries. These beneficial bacteria are very necessary to maintain a healthy balance in the gut, yet only about 25 percent of Americans have *Lactobacilli* species, compared with nearly 100 percent of the populations in Asia and Africa. The main reason for the lack of beneficial bacteria among Americans is *the Western diet*. Daily intake of probiotics in the form of supplements and selected foods can restore a healthy balance in your gut.

HOW DO PROBIOTICS WORK?

To understand how probiotics work in the body, it's important to know something about their work environment—the gut—how they get there, and what they are expected to do once they reach their destination. In order for probiotics to perform their various functions once they have been ingested, they must first successfully navigate through the high acidity (low pH) environment in the stomach and the bile salts in the small intestine. Not all beneficial bacteria or probiotics are able to survive this journey; some probiotic supplements and foods are not processed or stored properly for example, or they don't contain viable bacteria. That's why it's important that you take the correct and most stable microorganisms when choosing a probiotic supplement. (We help you make those choices in chapter 12.)

Once the probiotic microorganisms successfully reach the intestinal tract, they need to attach themselves to the intestinal, or mucosal, cells in the gut and begin to reproduce rapidly. They also become part of the bacterial flora that is already in your gut, both good and bad. The main function of the bacteria in your gut is to ferment dietary substances that your small intestine is not able to digest, including dietary fiber, proteins, oligosaccharides, and resistant starches. The average adult passes along about 800 grams (nearly two pounds) of food through the colon each day, and this food is partly processed by the bacteria through fermentation to produce lactic acid and short-chain fatty acids (SCFAs). These substances are primarily produced in the first section of the large intestine (ascending colon), while other factors (e.g., phenolic compounds, nitrogenous compounds) are produced further along in the intestinal tract (descending and sigmoid colon). Lactic acid is important in the production of probiotic foods such as yogurt, cheese, and sauerkraut, while SCFAs decrease the pH in the colon, improve absorption of calcium, iron, and magnesium, and provide energy to cells in the colon.

As you learned in this chapter, different species and strains of probiotics and other friendly bacteria each have their own beneficial characteristics; they inhabit certain areas of the gastrointestinal tract and target specific fats, proteins, and sugars for digestion. They also have one or more of the following properties—antimicrobial, anticancer, antidiarrheal, antioxidant, anti-inflammatory, and/or immune system modulator—and can deliver these benefits in a variety of ways. We talk about three of those ways below.

Fight Bad Bacteria

When you take probiotics on a daily basis, you replenish and restore your gut with beneficial microorganisms and allow them to establish themselves as a powerful good-bacteria force in your intestinal tract to fight against such serious pathogens as *Clostridia, Enterococcus, Escherichia coli, Salmonella, Shigella,* and *Pseudomonas,* and yeasts such as *Candida albicans.* Probiotics compete with the pathogens, engaging in a type of "turf war," and prevent them from colonizing in the gut, as well as battle the pathogens for nutrients that these disease-causing organisms need to survive. They also enhance the production of mucins, which help maintain a healthy mucosal barrier in the gut.

The ability of ingested probiotics to survive in different parts of the gut differs among the bacterial strains, which is one reason why it is important to take a variety of probiotic strains, as we discuss throughout this book. Research shows us that when probiotics are consumed daily, the beneficial bacteria can successfully colonize the intestinal tract rather quickly, within a few days. If you stop providing your body with good bacteria, however, the population of probiotics falls rapidly and an imbalance occurs.

Probiotics help normalize and balance beneficial flora in several ways. One way is through the secretion of antibacterial substances, including hydrogen peroxide, bacteriocins, and organic acids, which reduce the number of pathogens as well as hinder the production of toxins. Probiotics produce lactic acid, which results in a lowering of pH, thus improving the environment in the gut for the beneficial bacteria to grow and prosper.

Preserve Vitamins and Antioxidants

Probiotics regulate the metabolic activity of the bacterial flora in the gut. One way they do this is by reducing the pH in the intestinal tract, which then has a positive effect on the enzyme activity of the bacteria. Lactobacillus species are active in preserving vitamins and antioxidants, removing toxic food substances that can cause illness, and preventing activation of specific pathogens found in fermented foods (e.g., Enterobacteriacea, *S. aureus,* and Enterococci). Investigators have also found that *Bifidobacterium* strains can produce folate (folic acid), one of the essential B vitamins, and also help metabolize carbohydrates.

Several probiotics, specifically *Lactobacillus acidophilus, L. bulgaricus, Streptococcus thermophilus,* and *Bifidobacteria,* improve the digestion of lactose, breaking it down before it reaches the colon. This is important for people who are lactose intolerant (see more details about lactose intolerance in chapter 6). Some probiotics also have the ability to break down nitroamines, which are carcinogenic compounds that occur in certain acidic environments, such as in the stomach. This action is one way probiotics may help in the fight against cancer (see chapter 8 for more on probiotics and cancer).

Regulate the Immune System

Probiotics act as immunomodulators, which means they activate and regulate portions of the immune system in ways that can have a significant impact on various conditions associated with the immune system, including allergies and allergy-related diseases, inflammatory conditions such as arthritis, and the overall ability of the immune system to fight infection and disease. For example, probiotics help deliver anti-inflammatory molecules to the intestinal tract, enhance the ability of special host cells to reduce inflammation, and reduce inflammation by hindering the production of inflammatory substances. We discuss the benefits of probiotics in the immune system in much detail in chapter 8, and, specifically, their ability to impact asthma and allergies, in chapter 6.

BOTTOM LINE

In this chapter we introduced you to the many different species of beneficial bacteria that are important, not only to treat specific diseases and medical symptoms, but also to maintain health and well-being. You learned that different species of probiotics perform different tasks and can offer a variety of benefits. And we hope you come away with the fact that, while taking one species of probiotic is helpful, taking at least four or five provides you with a broader range of coverage against bad bacteria in your gut.

Probiotics have such a critical role in building and maintaining a strong foundation for health that they need to be supported and nurtured as much as possible. Substances that help probiotics perform their crucial work are the subject of the next chapter.

3

Prebiotics and
Other Probiotic Helpers

It's a tough world, and everyone—in fact, every living thing—can use a little help now and then to maneuver through the maze of life. Probiotics are no exception. That's why we need to introduce you to some very important little helpers for beneficial bacteria: prebiotics and enzymes.

A casual explanation of prebiotics is "it's the food probiotics eat," and since there are an enormous number of beneficial bacteria in the gut that need to be fed, a significant supply of quality prebiotics are needed not only to support them but to ensure their survival.

An official definition of prebiotics was assigned by the researchers who first identified them in 1995, but we'll skip the technical talk and get to the core of the matter. Prebiotics are carbohydrates, or more specifically, certain soluble (nondigestible) fibers that selectively stimulate the growth and/or activity of one or more species of bacteria in the colon and result in an improvement in health."

These fibers are present in whole foods, including selected vegetables, fruits, whole grains, and legumes, and they feed the *Bifidobacterium* species, which are the primary beneficial bacteria in the colon, but *Lactobacillus* species benefit as well. Prebiotics are very particular about which bacteria they team up with and affect. You might think of prebiotics as being like a special fertilizer for your garden, one that helps your flowers grow but that has no impact on the weeds.

Prebiotics help the beneficial bacteria survive their journey through the often hostile environment of the stomach and small intestine, and then support their growth and reproduction when they reach the gut. Once the probiotics reach their destination, with the help of prebiotics, they can then work to achieve the ultimate goal, which is to improve your health.

Characteristics of Prebiotics

We've already mentioned that not just any soluble fiber can be classified as a prebiotic: Only those soluble fibers that meet specific criteria qualify. Therefore, to be a prebiotic, a substance

- must not be digested or absorbed in the stomach or small intestine;
- must serve as the basis or foundation for growth or other activity for one or more beneficial bacteria;
- must be capable of modifying the bacterial flora in the gut toward a more balanced, healthy state; and
- must promote or induce beneficial systemic effects to the body.

Most of the soluble fibers that meet these requirements are members of a category of substances called oligosaccharides, a type of glycoside (sugar). They are found naturally in cereals and most plants, and are especially plentiful in artichokes, barley, beans and legumes, chicory, dandelion greens, eggplant, flax, garlic, leeks, onions, peas, and whole grains. (See chapter 12 for prebiotic foods and how to use them.)

The oligosaccharides most often used as prebiotic supplements in the United States are fructooligosaccharides (FOS) and inulins. FOS and inulins are natural sugars that are credited with providing various health benefits, including lowering triglyceride and cholesterol levels, stabilizing blood sugar, improving absorption of certain minerals, and improving insulin response, although much research is still needed in these areas. Let's examine these oligosaccharides.

Fructooligosaccharides

Fructooligosaccharides (FOS), also called neosugar, are the most abundant type of oligosaccharide. FOS are ideal prebiotics because they reach the large intestine virtually untouched, as humans do not have the enzymes that are needed to metabolize them. Therefore, the beneficial bacteria in the gut can utilize (ferment) FOS completely. FOS promote growth of beneficial bacteria in the gut, and especially stimulate the production and growth of *Bifidobacterium* species in the colon, where they can act as a strong barrier against disease-causing organisms. The addition of FOS to your diet can help relieve constipation and prevent the production of substances that degrade and damage proteins in the gut.

The standard American diet is low in FOS. Americans typically consume an average of 2.5 grams per day of this beneficial nutrient, compared with 12 to 18 grams daily consumed by people who eat a Mediterranean-type diet. Archaeologists who study the diets of our ancestors believe that our predecessors also consumed healthy amounts of prebiotics, especially those people who slow roasted root vegetables in earth ovens, a process that helped preserve inulin molecules. In fact, slow cooking is now recognized as one of the healthiest ways to prepare foods.

FOS are available as a dietary supplement alone, are added to some probiotic supplements, and are added to some functional foods by food manufacturers. They are also found naturally in certain foods, including asparagus, artichokes, bananas, chicory, garlic, leeks, onions, and wheat (see chapter 12 for a detailed look at prebiotic foods).

Inulins

Inulins belong to a class of carbohydrates called fructans. These prebiotics are found in or are derived from many of the same sources in which FOS are found. Food manufacturers also add inulins to many of their products because these fructans are sweet and have a pleasing texture. When you consider food sources and what is available as food additives, Americans consume about 1 to 4 grams of inulins per day, while Europeans get up to 10 grams.

Like FOS, inulins stimulate the production and growth of beneficial bacteria in the gut, especially *Bifidobacterium* species, and provide other health benefits, as outlined under "Prebiotics at Work." Inulins are available as a dietary supplement alone and with probiotics (see chapter 12).

Lactulose

Lactulose is a semisynthetic prebiotic that is composed of galactose and fructose. It is not found naturally. Lactulose has been used successfully in both animals and humans to reduce the growth and transmission of bad bacteria, especially *Salmonella.* In the United States, lactulose is a prescription drug used to treat constipation and hepatic encephalopathy, and it also appears to help relieve symptoms of inflammatory bowel disease. Some research also indicates that among postmenopausal women, lactulose stimulates the absorption of magnesium, and that it may also help people who have diabetes by improving glucose tolerance and carbohydrate metabolism. In Japan, lactulose is used as a nutritional supplement and in functional foods (foods that have demonstrated some physiological benefits and/or reduce the risk of chronic disease beyond the scope of basic nutrition).

Other Oligosaccharides

Other oligosaccharides include oligofructose, isomalto-oligosaccharides, lactosucrose, pyrodextrins, soy oligosaccharides, transgalacto-oligosaccharides, and xylo-oligosaccharides. (These are a mouthful to pronounce, but you may see them listed on your supplement labels.) All stimulate growth of *Bifidobacterium* species, and isomalto-oligosaccharides also promote growth of *Lactobacillus* species. These oligosaccharides are currently widely used in Japan as prebiotic supplements and in "functional foods," and they are also currently being developed in the United States for the same purposes.

Indeed, a review in 2006 of the use and effectiveness of prebiotics as a way to balance the flora in the gut showed that three prebiotics in particular—oligofructose, galacto-oligosaccharides, and lactulose—increase the levels of *Bifidobacterium* and *Lactobacillus* species in the gut. So far, they appear to help increase calcium absorption and to reduce inflammation in inflammatory bowel disease. Although studies of the benefits of prebiotics in people are in short supply, the findings obtained from the research that has been done thus far is very promising and offers plenty of reasons to include these healing substances in your daily diet.

PREBIOTICS AT WORK

Research indicates that prebiotics perform very critical functions once they are ingested and reach their destination, the large intestine. This is where they meet up and interact with beneficial bacteria, primarily *Bifidobacterium*, and to a lesser extent, *Lactobacillus* and other bacteria, to produce short-chain fatty acids (including propionate and butyrate), gases, and several other substances. Studies also show that FOS and other prebiotics display some very notable abilities once they are in the gut; namely, they can be anticarcinogens, antimicrobials, lipid-lowering agents (reduce cholesterol), glucose moderators (lower blood sugar levels), and antiosteoporotics (help prevent bone loss), as well as facilitators for the absorption of certain minerals. Prebiotics can perform these functions either alone and/or to assist the probiotics that also engage in these activities. Let's look at each of these possibilities individually. Some of the information is technical, but I believe you will also find it fascinating that so many factors in the food we eat and supplements we take can have such a positive and important impact on health.

Anticarcinogens

The possible anticarcinogenic actions of prebiotics may be partly attributed to butyrate, one of the short-chain fatty acids that is produced as a by-product of the bacterial fermentation that occurs between prebiotics and probiotics when they meet in the colon. Butyrate's anticancer activities may include the ability to increase programmed cell death, which means damaged and mutated cells (e.g., cancer cells) are destroyed more rapidly. The fatty acid may also help stop cell growth and cell differentiation, which are characteristic of cancer.

Apart from butyrate, prebiotics may also show some anticancer effects by increasing the concentrations of calcium in the colon, which may help control the formation of substances (salts of fatty acids and insoluble bile) that can damage colon cells and lead to the development of cancer. Several animal and lab studies have suggested that prebiotics can indirectly prevent the growth of tumors, inhibit the conversion of precarcinogens into carcinogens by some bacteria, and directly inactivate some carcinogens by binding with them.

Antimicrobials

Prebiotics are especially useful for promoting the growth and development of *Bifidobacterium* and *Lactobacillus* species in the gut. Once FOS and other prebiotics reach the gut and undergo fermentation, one result of this action is a significant reduction in the pH (or, if you prefer, an increase in acidity) in the intestinal tract. This change in the environment of the gut then leads to a reduction in the populations of disease-causing microorganisms, especially *Clostridia, E. coli, Klebsiella,* and *Enterobacter.* FOS and other prebiotics also help prevent unfriendly bacteria from attaching themselves to the gut wall and attempt to crowd the pathogens out of the gut. It is also believed that prebiotics produce antimicrobial substances and stimulate positive immune responses.

Butyrate has an antimicrobial role here, as it provides 70 percent of the energy for cells that are essential for the health of the intestinal tract. If butyrate levels are inadequate, these cells become unable to protect the mucosal barrier in the gut, and unfriendly bacteria and other pathogens can take over and tip the balance in a negative direction.

Lipid-Lowering Agents

Several studies with rats showed that prebiotics reduced triglyceride and cholesterol levels, and then subsequent animal studies revealed that blood insulin levels also declined significantly when FOS was administered. All of these findings were especially interesting because of the association between high cholesterol and triglycerides and diabetes, which is at epidemic levels. The reasons for the declines in triglycerides and cholesterol are not clear. One theory is that the prebiotics indirectly cause a decline in the synthesis of triglycerides. Another idea is that propionate, a by-product of fermentation in the colon, may inhibit the activity of the enzyme HMG-CoA reductase, which helps regulate the rate of cholesterol synthesis.

To see what effect FOS has on insulin, researchers conducted a double-blind, placebo-controlled trial in fifty-four middle-aged women and men who received 10 grams of FOS or placebo daily for eight weeks. At the end of the trial, insulin levels were significantly lower in the subjects who had taken FOS than in controls, and triglyceride levels were also markedly reduced.

Both animal and human studies indicate that inulins can lower total cholesterol and triglyceride levels. In one small double-blind, placebo-controlled, crossover study, for example, eight healthy men who were on a high-carbohydrate, low-fat diet were given inulins to see if and how they affected cholesterol and triglyceride levels. Triglyceride concentration levels and the liver's fat production were both substantially reduced, supporting the use of inulins to help reduce risk factors for atherosclerosis and heart disease.

Absorption Enhancers

Prebiotics also have the ability to decrease the pH in the colon, which makes the intestinal environment much more hospitable for probiotics and other beneficial bacteria to thrive and to absorb any calcium, as well as other minerals such as magnesium, and zinc, that remains in the food that has reached the colon. This feature makes prebiotics attractive as a way to possibly increase bone density and thus reduce the risk of osteoporosis and/or bone fractures.

Studies of calcium absorption have shown some impressive figures. In several rat studies, animals who were given 5% FOS had a 60 to 65 percent increase in calcium absorption. Rats in other studies had a reduction in the loss of calcium and phosphate from their bones.

Absorption rates in human volunteers were also significant. Adolescents who were given 5 grams of FOS daily had a 26 percent increase in calcium absorption, while adolescents in another study who took 8 grams per day had a 20 percent increase in absorption. (The difference in absorption between the two groups may have been related to other dietary factors.) The increase in calcium absorption may be the result of the oligosaccharides binding with the mineral in the small intestine, causing the short-chain fatty acids that form during fermentation to stimulate absorption.

Magnesium also gets a boost from prebiotics. In a study of postmenopausal women, those who consumed 10 grams of FOS daily had a 12 percent increase in magnesium absorption.

Blood Sugar Moderator

The ability of prebiotics to help regulate and balance blood sugar levels is a health benefit for everyone, but especially if you have prediabetes or diabetes. Experts do not yet fully understand how prebiotics provide this benefit, but one explanation is that they help slow the release of food from the stomach and/or the small intestine, which in turn moderates the amount of sugar in the bloodstream and the volume of insulin needed to transport it into the cells. This is an area that requires much more study.

Probiotics and Helpers Together

Ideally, you should include prebiotics, enzymes, and probiotics in your diet every day and at every meal, as food, supplements, or both.

Some single foods and common food combinations contain both pre- and probiotics and are referred to as *synbiotic* foods. Similarly, some probiotic supplements also contain prebiotics and thus are synbiotic as well. In chapter 12, we show you how easy it is to make probiotics, prebiotics, and enzymes a part of your lifestyle.

The precautions for prebiotics are similar to those for probiotics (see chapter 2). Information on how to purchase and use prebiotics is covered in chapter 12.

ENZYMES

Enzymes are proteins that make things happen: They are catalysts that initiate a wide spectrum of essential biochemical reactions—more than seven thousand—throughout the body, and in the process are not used up or altered chemically in any way. That means they can be used again and again to make chemical reactions occur in the body. If you didn't have enzymes, these biochemical reactions would happen very slowly or not at all, which in many cases would cause serious and even deadly results.

Because enzymes are proteins, they are composed of amino acids. The amino acid pattern is unique to each type of enzyme and gives the enzyme its own special function. If the specific pattern of an enzyme is altered or destroyed—many medications, other drugs, and chemicals damage or destroy enzymes—the enzyme can no longer perform its inherent tasks.

Why Talk About Enzymes?

The tasks of certain enzymes involve helping probiotics and prebiotics perform their functions. As we discussed at the beginning of chapter 2, some of the functions performed by probiotics include aiding digestion, assisting in the absorption of nutrients, producing vitamins, and enhancing calcium metabolism—all essential activities for life. Without the help of enzymes, these functions could not be completed. Therefore, here we examine a category of enzymes—digestive enzymes—which consists of substances that perform crucial digestive and metabolic activities that impact the ability of probiotics to do their job.

Another category, systemic enzymes, consists of substances that promote a wide variety of other functions throughout the body; for example, preventing tumor growth, fighting infections, assisting liver function and detoxification, reducing cholesterol buildup in the arteries, and stimulating immune system function. Probiotics need enzymes to complete these and other tasks in the body.

Digestive Enzymes

Digestive enzymes are important for digestion and overall health, and they support probiotic activity. Indeed, a combination of probiotic and digestive enzyme supplements is just the ticket for many people who suffer from a wide range of gastrointestinal disorders. From heartburn to gas to irritable bowel syndrome to colitis, gastrointestinal disorders are among the most common health complaints in the United States. One reason for these complaints is that the pancreas manufactures fewer and fewer digestive enzymes as you grow older. Indeed, the level of digestive enzymes declines sharply after age forty. When you combine this natural process with the fact that the standard American diet contains very low amounts of natural digestive enzymes from plant foods, you are left with an overall diet lacking in sufficient levels of enzymes to properly digest foods. A deficiency of enzymes also means nutrients are not made available to the probiotics and to the body.

You can improve your enzyme status by increasing your intake of foods that contain live enzymes (e.g., raw fruits and vegetables, sprouted legumes, and similar uncooked foods), taking enzyme supplements along with meals, or a combination of the two. I recommend the latter approach, because nothing can beat nature's enzymes! However, most people don't have the lifestyle or the desire to make dramatic changes in their diet, so a combination of enzyme supplements and more foods rich in live enzymes, is a wise choice. (We offer you dietary tips, food choices, and recipes in chapter 12.)

Various types of digestive enzymes that are important for digestion and overall health, and support probiotic activity, are available as supplements, typically as a combination product. When shopping for enzyme supplements, look for products that provide a variety of digestive enzymes, like those listed below. (See chapter 12 for more information on how to purchase enzymes.)

- *Protease and peptidase.* Protease and peptidase are both proteolytic enzymes, which means they break down nonliving protein (proteins in food) while not harming living protein in the body's tissues. Protease enzymes digest protein molecules by breaking the peptide bonds that link the amino acids together. Peptidase then completes the digestion of protein. Therefore, both enzymes are necessary for protein metabolism to take place. *This is an important fact to remember, because enzyme supplements that supply one enzyme but not the other will not effectively digest protein.* (See chapter 12 for more information on enzyme supplements.) Both of these enzymes also can be categorized as systemic enzymes (see "Systemic Enzymes"), because they help prevent inflammation and accompanying pain by allowing the body to absorb renegade protein fragments that can accumulate in tissues and joints.

- *Amylase and alpha-galactosidase.* These enzymes help digest both simple and complex carbohydrates, but each one targets different types of carbs. Amylase works primarily on starches, breaking down complex carbs (polysaccharides) into very small units called monosaccharides, such as glucose. Alpha-galactosidase works on different carbohydrates (e.g., raffinose, verbascose) and also helps prevent the gas and bloating that often occur after you eat high-fiber foods such as beans.

- *Glucoamylase, invertase, and malt diastase.* Each of these enzymes works on digesting sugars, but each has its own specialty. Glucoamylase breaks down polysaccharides; invertase focuses on sucrose; while malt diastase works on maltose and breaks it down to glucose.

- *Lipase and lipase AN.* These enzymes help digest fats and oils. The liver begins the process by emulsifying large fat molecules, and then the bile breaks them down to smaller fragments, which the lipase and lipase AN can digest. When fats and oils are not metabolized properly, they can cause weight gain, high blood pressure, and high cholesterol.

- *Cellulase and pectinase.* Cellulase breaks down cellulose, the indigestible fiber found in fruits and vegetables, while pectinase focuses on pectin, a carbohydrate found in fruits. Both of these enzymes also assist in bowel regularity.

- *Phytase, hemicullulase, and xylanase.* These three enzymes break down carbohydrates that are found in plants as well as the fiber in the vegetables. Phytase also has another function: increasing the bioavailability and absorption of calcium, iron, magnesium, and zinc in the body, all important in the fight against bone density loss.

- *Lactase.* If you need help digesting milk and milk products, lactase is the enzyme you would enlist for help. Lactase breaks down lactose, the main sugar found in milk from cows and other mammals, into two simple sugars.

Systemic Enzymes

Systemic enzymes circulate throughout the body and perform vital functions other than digestive activities, such as fighting viruses, reducing inflammation, digesting scar tissue, regulating the immune system, and cleansing the blood. Despite their importance in supporting and maintaining health, systemic enzymes are usually ignored or overlooked by physicians in the United States. In other countries, and especially in Germany, they are widely used to treat pain and inflammation and for heart health, the immune system, and sports injuries.

Similar to digestive enzymes, which have an appetite for proteins, fats, and carbohydrates, systemic enzymes have an appetite for specific substances as well. Among the systemic enzymes that cleanse the blood, for example, some break down fibrin, which helps reduce the formation of blood clots and thus minimizes the risk of stroke and heart attack. Other enzymes digest dead cells so they can be eliminated more easily in the bowel.

Unlike digestive enzymes, which do not need to be absorbed by the body to complete their tasks, systemic enzymes need to get into the bloodstream and be carried to locations throughout the body to perform their various functions. That's why systemic enzymes are taken on an empty stomach, between meals, which helps them enter the bloodstream efficiently. You will notice that several of the enzymes we discuss—proteases and peptidases in particular—can be classified as both digestive and systemic enzymes. However, when they are taken with meals, they act as digestive enzymes; when taken between meals, they perform systemic functions.

Supplements of several systemic enzymes can be especially helpful in treating certain symptoms and diseases when they are taken along with probiotics. For individuals who have an upper respiratory tract infection, for example, I often recommend systemic enzymes, along with a probiotic program, because of the ability of these enzymes to fight inflammation and regulate the immune system (see chapter 6).

The types of systemic enzymes I typically recommend are protease and peptidase enzymes, which we discussed in the section on digestive enzymes; and bromelain, which, like protease and peptidase enzymes, also acts as both a systemic and digestive enzyme (see "Digestive Enzymes").

Bromelain is a mixture of sulfur-containing, protein-eating enzymes that is found in the stem of pineapples (*Ananas comosus*). When taken in between meals or on an empty stomach, it is especially efficient at reducing inflammation that is associated with physical injuries and infections, such as upper respiratory tract infections and urinary tract infections. It is not known as a great digestive enzyme. If you are an athlete or are physically active, bromelain should be a part of your daily supplement program.

Benefits of Systemic Enzymes

- **Fight inflammation.** Systemic enzymes such as proteases, bromelain, and papain digest a damaging type of proteins called Circulating Immune Complexes, which are a leading cause of inflammation and joint pain.
- **Fight viruses.** Enzymes digest the outer protein coating on viruses, which then may make it impossible for them to attach themselves to your cells' DNA and reproduce.

continued

Box continued

- **Digest scar tissue and fibrosis.** As you age, your supply of enzymes declines, which leaves fewer enzymes to help eliminate the fibrin and scar tissue that builds up throughout the body. Uterine fibroids, endometriosis, and fibrocystic breast are examples of conditions in which fibrin has accumulated in the body. Scar tissue also accumulates in blood vessels and organs, jeopardizing their function. When you replace lost enzymes, you can help control and reduce the amount of fibrosis that occurs in the body.
- **Regulate the immune system.** Enzymes "sense" how the immune system is functioning and can help balance it. If you are experiencing inflammation from, let's say, arthritis or lupus, your immune system is overactive. Enzymes can digest excess antibodies that are damaging your immune system. Similarly, if your immune system is underactive (e.g., you have an infection), enzymes can boost white blood cell and natural killer cell activity and help fight the illness.
- **Cleanse the blood.** Systemic enzymes can be counted on to remove excess fibrin from the blood, which helps reduce the formation of blood clots, and thus minimizes the risk of stroke and heart attack. Some enzymes are responsible for breaking down dead cells and other material so it can be eliminated in the bowel. These and other cleansing functions help take stress off the liver, which is the body's primary filtering/cleansing organ.

Papain is derived from unripe papaya (pawpaw). Along with its digestive benefits, papain helps eliminate parasites in the gut by digesting them, and also cleans up dead cellular materials in the bloodstream. Papain and bromelain are often available in a combination supplement.

Coenzymes and Other Helpers

You already know that enzymes help probiotics, but what happens when enzymes need help in order to support the probiotics? That's when you call in coenzymes. (For the record: a nonprotein helper of enzymes is called a cofactor; if the cofactor is organic, it is called a coenzyme. For simplicity's sake, we refer to both as "coenzymes.") Coenzymes are a smaller molecule compared with the protein part of an enzyme. Many different substances can serve as coenzymes, including vitamins, minerals, herbs, and proteins. Because the body consumes coenzymes all the time, they must be replaced regularly.

Among the coenzymes that are especially helpful when taking probiotics are calcium, manganese, zinc, and copper, all of which need to be taken in a highly bioavailable chelated form to be effective (look for a high-quality multimineral supplement). Calcium supplements help stop the loss of this critical mineral from the bones, while manganese works with various enzymes to facilitate dozens of different metabolic processes throughout the body. Supplementing with the coenzyme manganese is especially important for anyone who experiences inflammation and pain, because it is part of the antioxidant enzyme SOD (superoxide dismutase), which is also composed of zinc and copper. SOD relies on support from dietary (food and/or supplements) manganese, zinc, and copper to neutralize free radicals and thus help prevent inflammation.

Another helper I frequently recommend as part of a probiotic plan is MSM, or methylsulfonylmethane. MSM is a natural form of organic sulfur that helps enzymes function optimally, supports immune system functioning, promotes digestion, is a building block for proteins (for joints, skin, hair, nails, and cartilage), relieves inflammation and pain, helps heal the mucous membrane that lines the gut, and assists with circulation and nutrient absorption. It is found in very small amounts in fresh, raw foods, including fruits, vegetables, and grains, but it is easily depleted once these foods are processed or heated. Because the standard American diet consists largely of highly processed, cooked foods, this natural form of sulfur is lacking in most people's diets. Fortunately, MSM is also available as a dietary supplement.

Yet one more probiotic helper is sodium chlorite (NaClO2), sometimes referred to as stabilized oxygen. Sodium chlorite is a precursor to chlorine dioxide and consists of two oxygen molecules that are bonded to a chloride molecule. When sodium chlorite enters the body and encounters the pH, the two oxygen molecules break away from the chloride molecule and oxygenate the colon, which helps destroy yeast and support the beneficial bacteria. Thus sodium chlorite is useful as an antiviral, antifungal, and antibacterial agent that can support the elimination of yeast and other infections when taken internally. It is typically sold as a 5% solution that you add to water and drink (see chapter 12 for purchasing information).

BOTTOM LINE

The use of prebiotics, enzymes, and other probiotic helpers can significantly enhance the benefits of any probiotics you take. Prebiotics and enzymes can be found in many common foods and can easily be included in your daily diet. (See chapter 12 for tips and recipe ideas.) You also have the option of taking these probiotic helpers in the form of supplements. Either way, you can expect to experience a positive difference when you include prebiotics, enzymes, and other health enhancers as part of your dietary lifestyle.

PART II

Your Probiotic

Health Plan

4

The Core Program:

Build a Better You

Virtually every woman, man, and child can benefit from restoring and maintaining a balanced bacterial flora in the gut. Let's say you are already health-conscious and you and your family take a daily multivitamin supplement or individual nutrients, because you want to have a strong foundation to help avoid any potential health problems. Your efforts may be largely wasted, unless your body is in a state of health to efficiently accept and use all the nutrients you send its way. You need a balanced bacterial environment in your gut to help you fight off unfriendly bacteria and other pathogens and to get the most benefit from your nutrients. The bottom line is quite simple: It doesn't matter how healthful your diet is or how many supplements you take; if your bacterial flora is out of balance, you cannot enjoy good health.

That's why we begin our discussion of probiotic health plans with a simple core program that is designed to enhance energy, vitality, and well-being and protect against everyday stressors. We hope you incorporate these guidelines and the probiotic health plan—both of which are provided at the end of this chapter—into your lifestyle. In the chapters that follow, we'll focus on specific health problems that can be treated effectively with probiotics.

WHO CAN BENEFIT FROM A PROBIOTICS HEALTH PROGRAM

Frank is a thirty-four-year-old computer programmer who says he feels "about average." "I'm relatively fit, and I'd say I have a regular amount of energy, although I could use some more. I don't get much planned exercise, but I work around the house and the yard on weekends and take the dog for a walk when the kids forget. I don't have any health problems per se—no chronic illness, no significant aches or pains. I don't smoke, but I like to kick back with a few beers on weekends and sometimes some wine during the week. I know I eat too much fast food, but my wife and I eat healthier at home. Sometimes I get really sleepy at work, and I try to catch up on my sleep on weekends."

Connie, a twenty-nine-year-old single mother, admits she could stand to lose about twenty pounds, but she says she feels "pretty good" most of the time. "My two kids keep me busy," she says, "and I work part-time as a hair stylist, so I'm on my feet a lot. I don't worry too much about the chemicals I'm exposed to at work, although I guess I should. Getting enough sleep is always a problem. I don't smoke or drink, and I try to make good meals at home most of the time because I want my kids to grow up healthy. But we do eat at fast-food restaurants probably more than we should."

Margaret is a recently retired teacher who is trying to adjust to her new lifestyle. "I'm looking forward to traveling and volunteering with my church, and I want to take some classes in pottery making," she says. "I want to make sure I have the energy to do all these things.

Fortunately I'm in pretty good health, just a little arthritis and my blood pressure is a bit high, but I take medication for it. I know I need to eat better, and I plan to make that a priority."

Frank, Connie, and Margaret are "okay," but all of them could benefit from a healthier lifestyle, including a balanced environment in their gut. They, like so many Americans, are exposed to or experience daily, often insidious assaults to their health and well-being that will likely develop into a significant, chronic, or even life-threatening problem some day—a problem such as diabetes, heart disease, cancer, stroke, fibromyalgia, irritable bowel disease, chronic fatigue syndrome, obesity, or osteoporosis. And then there is the one condition that affects everyone: aging, and all the changes that accompany that transformation.

People of all ages come to me constantly, asking how they can get healthy. When I take a blood sample and examine it, I see colonies of bacteria that are having a negative impact on their health. We discuss the benefits of probiotics and enzymes, and in most cases they start taking the supplements. After about a month, some people come back with a strange tale: They tell me they are getting results, they feel much better, but they think they had better stop the supplements. Why? Because they used to have a bowel movement every two to three days, and now they have one daily—and it's "inconvenient."

A healthy intestinal track and digestive system eliminates waste every day. The "inconvenience" these clients complain about is a healthy activity that they have not experienced before. Part of building a better you is having daily bowel movements and helping your body rid itself of toxins. That buildup is also about eating nutritious food, managing stress, avoiding environmental toxins, and maintaining a healthy bacterial flora in your intestinal tract. Health is not inconvenient, being unhealthy is.

Can your habits and lifestyle choices really have a significant impact on the critical beneficial bacterial balance in your gut? Definitely, and here's how.

POOR DIETARY HABITS

The relationship between poor diet and nutritional deficiencies and compromised intestinal health is clear: Beneficial bacteria and probiotics need the right food to develop, reproduce, and perform their many functions. If they are deprived of this basic need, the bad bacteria will thrive and keep the bacterial flora in their favor—to your detriment. The best foods to promote probiotics and friendly bacteria are fermented foods (e.g., yogurt, tempeh, sauerkraut, pickled vegetables), complex carbohydrates (e.g., whole grains, fresh fruits and vegetables, legumes and beans) and generally, foods that are low in bad fats and sugars. Fast food, fried foods, refined and processed foods, sugar, alcohol, and animal fats all promote the growth and development of bad bacteria. A change in dietary habits also means a change for the better in terms of intestinal health, and thus overall health as well.

The fact that beneficial bacteria need foods that have a certain chemical makeup while bad bacteria and yeasts thrive on other types of foods is basic biochemistry, and an interesting condition to explore. That's why researchers conduct studies like the one in which investigators deprived healthy volunteers of their normal fare of fermented foods (e.g., yogurt). Within two weeks, all the volunteers had a significant drop in their levels of beneficial lactobacillus and short-chain fatty acids, which placed them all in jeopardy of being unable to fight off infections. The volunteers were then given either probiotic supplements (containing *L. gasseri* and *L. coryniformis*) or were allowed to resume eating yogurt, which contained *L. delbrueckii* sp. *bulgaricus*. Both the yogurt and the supplement greatly improved the levels of beneficial bacteria, although the supplement was more effective than the yogurt.

Because the relationship between nutrition and gut health is so critical, we return to the topic throughout this book, but especially in two chapters: In chapter 5 we discuss probiotics and gastrointestinal disorders, and again in chapter 12, where we offer you tips and delicious, easy ways to incorporate probiotics and their helpers into your diet. Please turn to those chapters for more information.

LACK OF SLEEP

Before the lightbulb was invented, Americans slept an average of 10 hours per night. Now they sleep an average of 6.9 hours on weeknights and 7.5 hours on weekends. Although the availability of reliable artificial light may have made us less likely to go to bed early, did it also change how much sleep we *need*?

The answer, of course, is no, but that doesn't change the fact that too many people don't get enough sleep. In fact, many adults are sleeping only 4 to 5 hours per night. "Enough" is usually defined as at least eight hours of quality, continuous sleep (bathroom breaks don't count), although some people need as many as 10 hours. You can get a good idea whether you are getting enough sleep by answering the questions in the section, "Are You Sleep Deprived?" Answer the questions honestly, because even though you may not realize it, sleep deprivation takes its toll, often unnoticed, until it "catches up with you." And much of that toll begins in your gut.

Sleep, Bacteria, and Your Gut

What's the connection between bacteria in your gut and how much sleep you get? The microorganisms in your gut are directly influenced by your circadian rhythms, which are the regular physical and mental changes that occur during a twenty-four-hour period. These rhythms impact many of your activities, including your sleep/wake cycle, appetite and eating, and hormone production.

Most circadian rhythms are controlled by a miniscule part of the brain called the suprachiastmatic nucleus (SCN), better known as the "biological clock." During the day, light enters the eye, reaches the retina, and send signals to the SCN, which sends messages to the pineal gland. This gland switches off production of the hormone melatonin, and that switching off helps you stay alert. As darkness approaches, melatonin production gears up and increases, making you feel sleepy. Sleep and darkness melatonin promote activity of white blood cells, which fight unfriendly bacteria in the gut, and increase production of T cells and natural killer cells, which also help destroy harmful gut flora. If you don't get enough sleep, you shortchange the critical bacteria rebalancing activity in your gut. Sleep loss is also associated with an increase in factors that cause inflammation (e.g., C-reactive protein), which have a negative impact on the development and severity of heart disease.

Thus, the bacteria in your gut have a lifestyle that goes something like this: During the day they feast on available food (sugars and carbohydrates for the bad bacteria, fiber and other prebiotics for the good bacteria), and at night, with sleep, much of the fighting goes on as the immune system is triggered to destroy harmful bacteria and other pathogens. The bottom line is that you need an adequate amount of sleep to allow your beneficial bacteria to work toward a balanced, healthy environment in your gut.

Are You Sleep Deprived?

Here are some signs that you are sleep deprived. Do you

- need an alarm clock to wake up in the morning?
- fall asleep within five minutes of your head hitting the pillow? People who are well rested usually don't fall asleep for at least ten minutes after lying down
- nap easily?
- have difficulty concentrating during the day?
- feel groggy in the morning after waking up?
- often feel drowsy or tired during the day?
- easily fall asleep when you sit down to watch television?
- easily fall asleep when you sit down and read?
- experience feelings of anxiety, depression, irritability, or moodiness?
- doze off when you are a passenger in a car for an hour or longer without a break?

Sleep deprivation, or sleep debt, can occur after just one night of poor sleep or be the result of several days of poor sleep. The good news is that you can "make up" your sleep debt by getting some extra sleep a few nights in a row, but if you are chronically in sleep deprivation, your body will not be able to catch up and your health can suffer.

Here are some sleep and sleep deprivation facts. Are you or your family members part of these statistics?

- Nearly 70 percent of Americans report having frequent sleep problems.
- Ten to 15 percent of Americans have chronic and/or severe insomnia (NIH).
- About 47 million adults are at risk for health, injury, and behavior

difficulties because they don't get the minimum amount of sleep required to be alert during the day.

- Sleep deprivation is not limited to adults: 69 percent of children experience sleep problems at least a few nights per week.

- About 56,000 motor vehicle crashes per year are associated with driver drowsiness or fatigue, according to the National Highway Traffic Safety Administration. Roughly 1,550 deaths per year result from these crashes.

- The National Sleep Foundation reports that in their 2002 poll, 51 percent of Americans said they drove while feeling sleepy in the past year, and 17 percent dozed off while driving.

Sunlight: The Other Side of Darkness

Because your intestinal microorganisms are so influenced by your circadian rhythms, it is important to also mention, along with the importance of sleep, how exposure to sunlight is also important for intestinal health. In fact, sunlight is critical for your gut for several reasons.

One reason is for balance. A healthy circadian rhythm requires a balanced cycle of melatonin. As we mentioned, this hormone's production increases at night and decreases during daylight, and this natural rhythm is necessary for the beneficial bacteria in your gut to function optimally.

Another reason sunlight is important concerns vitamin D. Daily exposure to direct sunlight (without the use of sunscreen) for five to fifteen minutes between the hours of 10 AM and 3 PM during autumn, spring, and summer is enough for most people to produce vitamin D. (If you plan to stay out in the sun any longer, you should apply sunscreen.) How is the intestinal tract involved with vitamin D? The gut is one of the major destinations of vitamin D, where it regulates calcium metabolism, which is critical for bone health and many other functions.

STRESS

Do you ever get butterflies in your stomach? Do you experience diarrhea or stomach pain when you are in a tense, emotional, or stressful situation? Then you are familiar with what can happen when the relationship between the brain and the gut—the brain-gut axis as we discussed in chapter 1—is challenged, in this case by stress.

Stress has a significant impact on your gut. We know, for example, that chronic stress is a major factor in the development of irritable bowel syndrome and in the worsening of symptoms of Crohn's disease, ulcerative colitis, and other inflammatory conditions of the bowel. Stress also causes the gut to become hypersensitive, which makes some people develop allergies to certain foods.

Specifically, we know that chronic psychological stress causes the protective mucosal barrier in the intestinal tract to become less effective at defending the body against unfriendly bacteria and other disease-causing organisms.

Can probiotics help protect that barrier? Scientists in Canada wanted to find out, so they studied three groups of rats: One group was subjected to chronic psychological stress, and this group was divided in half—half received probiotics in their drinking water and the other half did not. The third group of rats served as a control group.

The scientists designed the stress sessions to mimic stress that would produce the type of responses seen in the human gut. At the end of the ten-day test period, the investigators found that most of the chronically stressed rats who did not receive probiotics had experienced a breakdown in their immune response—that is, bad bacteria had traveled to their mesenteric lymph nodes. This is an indication that the bacteria had come from the intestinal tract. Among the rats who received probiotics, however, there was nearly no sign of bacteria in the lymph nodes. This finding was an indication to the scientists that probiotics can prevent stress-induced damage to the intestinal tract and thus help maintain the health of the immune system.

DRINKING FOR HEALTH

Chlorinated water, alcohol, and coffee all have a detrimental effect on the bacterial flora in your gut. Chlorinated water not only kills beneficial bacteria in the intestinal tract, it also contains carcinogens known as trihalomethanes, which accumulate in the fatty tissues of the body and can cause cell mutation and suppress immune system function. Chlorinated water also aggravates asthma, especially in children who are exposed to chlorinated swimming pools, and it has been linked with a greater incidence of bladder and other cancers.

Coffee can have two effects on intestinal health. While the caffeine in coffee (and in tea and colas) can act as a laxative, coffee and other caffeine-containing beverages also are diuretics, which remove fluids from the body and can cause constipation.

When it comes to alcohol and the gut, moderation is the key. Excessive alcohol use, however, in addition to being toxic to the entire body, can reduce the ability of the intestines to contract and transport fecal material, which can then lead to toxic bacterial growth and disease.

USE OF ANTIBIOTICS

The introduction of antibiotics to the medical scene in the early twentieth century was eventually hailed as a turning point in health care.

Certainly much good has come out of Alexander Fleming's rediscovery of penicillin in 1928 (penicillin was originally noticed by Ernest Duchesne, a French medical student, in 1896) and its eventual use for the public in the 1940s, when Howard Florey and Ernst Chain isolated the active ingredient and produced a penicillin powder.

But misuse and too much of a good thing can have negative consequences, and antibiotic use is an excellent example of that turn. When you take antibiotics, they kill not only the disease-causing bacteria but the friendly ones as well. This throws your intestinal flora into a headspin, and the bad bacteria come out ahead and typically cause diarrhea. Antibiotic use can also cause yeast infections (e.g., a *Candida albicans* infection) to take hold, because the unbalanced gut environment is a welcome place for such an infection to occur, and yeast cells are immune to the effects of antibiotics. Once a *Candida albicans* infection becomes established, it takes some time to eliminate it (see chapter 7).

Even one course of antibiotics (and this includes all types of antibiotics, including aminoglycosides, cephalosporins, macrolides, quinolones, and tetracyclines) can cause serious damage to your gut health, and so they should be used only after other viable alternatives have been eliminated. The longer you take antibiotics, the more likely you are to develop a *Candida albicans* infection. Another infection, *Clostridium difficile,* is a common side effect of antibiotic use in the elderly. To help prevent these and other harmful effects from antibiotic treatment, you should take high doses of probiotics before, during, and after antibiotic treatment (see "Core Program" in this chapter).

Don't forget the antibiotics that are in your food. If you eat meat, poultry, fish, and dairy products from animals that have been raised conventionally, then you are getting antibiotics (along with hormones and various toxins) in every mouthful. These drugs, either alone or along with courses of antibiotic treatment, take their toll on the beneficial bacteria in your gut.

SMOKING

The relationship between smoking and lung cancer and other lung problems is well known, but the smoke doesn't stop in the lungs. When a smoker inhales, the smoke also enters the stomach and intestinal tract, where it has an impact on bacterial flora. This explains why smoking is associated with various gastrointestinal disorders and symptoms, including bloating, gas, abdominal pain and cramping, and why it causes or contributes to acid reflux (GERD), heartburn, Crohn's disease, and cancer of the stomach and esophagus.

Beneficial bacteria need the right food and the right environment in which to thrive. When you introduce nicotine and the more than 6,000 other chemicals found in cigarette smoke into the body, you can be sure they're up to no good, providing neither the right nourishment nor the right environment for probiotics and their helpers. Smoking, for example, generates high levels of free radicals, which deplete the body of disease-fighting antioxidants and nutrients needed by beneficial bacteria. Studies also show that chronic smoking can increase the amount of acid secreted by the stomach.

IMPORTANCE OF GOOD BOWEL HABITS

Before she began to take probiotics, Audrey had a common problem: Although she rated her health as "pretty good," she often experienced headaches, mild nausea, and even light-headedness whenever she had difficulty moving her bowels.

"I wasn't really constipated," she said, "just irregular. I normally move my bowels at least once a day; but several times a month, and at different times, I would miss a day, and then by the beginning of the third day I would have a headache and feel slightly nauseous and lightheaded. If I didn't go by the end of the day, I would take a laxative, and then I would go back to my normal pattern until it happened again. Taking laxatives was a habit I didn't want to get into, so I took a look at my eating habits and lifestyle, added probiotics, and within weeks I was regular again. Now I don't experience headaches or nausea and I'm a once-a-day gal again!"

By now you know just how important it is to your overall health to maintain a healthy balance of bacteria in your intestinal tract. That balance is in jeopardy whenever fecal matter remains in the bowels for days. Although some experts explain that having a bowel movement every three to four days is "normal" for some people, it is not healthy.

- Establish a "best time" of the day to have a bowel movement. Many people find that thirty to sixty minutes after a meal (usually breakfast) is the best, because that's when the body uses the gastro-colic reflex, which is a bowel motion that automatically occurs when you eat. This reflex helps produce a bowel movement. This is the body's natural way to say "it's time to get things moving!"
- Allow yourself some quiet, unrushed time to use the bathroom.
- Don't delay: When you have to go, heed the call. If you put it off, you risk experiencing hard, dry stools.
- Don't strain; this can lead to the development of hemorrhoids.
- The bowel is an organ of habit, it functions best when it receives roughly the same amount of food at each meal. That is, the amount of food you always eat at breakfast should be similar, and so on. It does *not* mean you need to eat the same amount of food at breakfast, lunch, and dinner.
- Eat your meals at a regular time each day.
- Eat enough fiber (25–30 grams per day) every day. If you include

prebiotic foods and supplements in your diet, this should be easy! (See chapter 12.)

- Drink about 64 ounces of noncaffeinated fluids daily. Caffeine draws fluid from the colon and can result in hard stools.
- Participate in daily exercise, and try to do it at the same time each day. "If I don't take my morning walk, I'm almost guaranteed to become irregular," says Bettina, a fifty-two-year-old medical office secretary. "If I can't walk in the morning before work, I make sure I walk before I eat lunch."
- Get into a good toilet position. Yes, there is one! Sit on the toilet, lean forward, and place your forearms on your thighs. Keep your back straight, and raise your feet (on a footstool) so your legs are angled slightly upward.

THE CORE PROGRAM

If your mother was like mine, she was always reminding you to eat your vegetables. Now we know just how right Mom was about that nutritional advice. If she had known about probiotics, she probably would have told us to eat them, too, and for good reason: They can help keep the bacterial flora in your gut in balance.

So here is the equivalent of your mother telling you to eat your veggies, except you don't have to eat broccoli and lima beans if you don't want to (but it's not a bad idea!). The recommended core probiotic supplement program is simple: Take a supplement that contains at least 2 billion colony-forming units (CFUs) representing as many different stabilized probiotic species as possible. In other words, if you have a choice between a probiotic supplement that contains *L. acidophilus* and *B. bifidum* alone and one that contains *L. acidophilus* DDS-1 as well as

L. casei, B. bifidum, B. longum, and *S. thermophilus,* choose the supplement that has five species. Here's why:

As you've learned so far, each species of beneficial bacteria/probiotic has its own specialty, strengths, and weaknesses. Some are better at eliminating certain bad bacteria than others; some stick to cell walls better or are very good at manufacturing B vitamins, while others are not. If you take only one or two species, you deprive yourself of the many benefits probiotics have to offer and don't provide your gut with all the ammunition it needs to battle the bad bacteria.

You don't need to depend solely on supplements to take advantage of beneficial bacteria; in fact, I strongly encourage you to incorporate probiotic foods in your diet daily—and at every meal if you can. (See chapter 12 for lots of tips and recipes concerning probiotic foods.) Consumption of a combination of probiotic foods and supplements daily can provide you with a solid foundation for health.

In addition, I urge you to evaluate your lifestyle and make positive changes in the areas we discussed above, all of which impact the balance of beneficial bacteria in your gut (see "Support Probiotics"). After all, while it's critical to include probiotics as part of your daily routine, just taking them isn't enough. You have to nurture and support them, too!

SUPPORT PROBIOTICS

These lifestyle tips are just a few examples of how you can nurture and support your probiotic program (which follows this list).

Diet
- Include prebiotic and probiotic foods in your diet every day, preferably at every meal. See chapter 12 for recipes and menu ideas.

- Avoid foods that support bad bacteria, e.g., foods that contain animal fat, foods made with white flour and/or sugar, fried foods, foods that contain preservatives, antibiotics, hormones, and other unnatural ingredients.
- Eat raw fruits and vegetables every day. They are a good source of enzymes, which support the work of probiotics.

Sleep

- Relax before bedtime. Engaging in exercise or stimulating physical or mental activities before going to bed can make it very difficult to fall asleep.
- Avoid caffeine and alcohol. (This tip is recommended for more than helping sleep!) Caffeine is a stimulant, and although alcohol initially acts as a sedative, it can interrupt normal sleep.
- Be wise about light and dark. When you wake up in the morning, expose yourself to sunlight or another source of bright light; when you sleep, keep your bedroom dark. These steps help regulate your circadian rhythm.

Stress

- Find enjoyable ways to manage stress and practice them daily. Examples include deep breathing, tai chi, yoga, meditation, massage, sauna, or taking time to read a favorite book or watch your favorite comedy tapes.
- Exercise regularly. Participating in enjoyable physical activities is a great stress reducer.

Drinking Habits

- Avoid chlorinated and fluoridated water. Instead, install a water filter in your home. In the long run, this approach is healthier, less expensive, and more environmentally responsible than buying bottled water.

- Choose healthy alternatives to coffee (e.g., herbal teas, grain beverages) and alcohol.

Smoking

- If you smoke, take advantage of any of the many programs or techniques available on how to quit.
- If you don't smoke but live with people who do, your health (and that of your children) is in jeopardy. If the smokers will not quit, make sure they do not smoke in the house or any vehicles or in the presence of family members.

Antibiotics

- If your doctor prescribes antibiotics for a bacterial infection, discuss possible alternative treatments.
- If antibiotics are necessary, make sure to take probiotics before, during, and after treatment (see chapter 8).

Here is a list of the stabilized probiotic species that I recommend. Your probiotic supplement should contain at least five of the twelve listed, but the more the better. You should get your probiotic supplements from a reputable manufacturer only (see chapter 12 for guidelines on buying probiotic, prebiotic, and enzyme supplements).

Stabilized Probiotic Species

L. acidophilus DDS-1 (this strain should be a part of
any probiotic program)

L. casei

L. plantarum

B. bifidum

B. longum

Bacillus coagulans

B. infantis

L. rhamnosus

L. salviarius

Lactococcus lactis

E. faecium

S. thermophilus

Core Program

- Take at least a total of 2 billion CFUs daily of five or more stabilized species/strains of beneficial bacteria. For children younger than ten years, 500 million to 1 billion is recommended.
- Take a probiotic supplement and/or eat probiotic food at each meal.
- Include a prebiotic supplement or food with each meal. Detailed information on different prebiotic foods and supplements, as well as recipes and menu ideas, are found in chapter 12.

PRECAUTIONS AND SIDE EFFECTS

Generally, probiotics are very safe and can be used by most adults and children without causing any significant discomfort or problems. The most common side effects are constipation and flatulence, which typically disappear within a few days as the gut adjusts to the introduction of friendly bacteria and the rebalancing of the bacterial flora. These temporary symptoms are akin to the dust you kick up when you do spring cleaning: Once the dust settles, you have a cleaner, more organized house. In rare cases, people are hypersensitive to some component(s) of a probiotic supplement. Make sure you read the label carefully before you take any probiotic supplement and look for those that have the fewest (or no) additives. (We discuss how to shop for probiotics in chapter 12.)

If you are pregnant or nursing, consult with your doctor before taking probiotic supplements. If you want to use probiotics to treat a medical condition, make sure your physician supervises your treatment. Also talk to your doctor before taking probiotics if you are elderly, or if you have a medical condition that significantly compromises your immune system (e.g., HIV, AIDS, organ transplant, kidney or liver disease). If you cannot digest milk-based products or if you are a vegan (you choose not to consume milk products), you should know there are virtually no milk products in probiotic supplements.

BOTTOM LINE

Good health and well-being depend on regular restoration of the beneficial flora in your gut. For many people, simply introducing probiotics at each meal, as a supplement and/or food, goes a long way toward achieving this goal and is the foundation of a basic healthful life program. This approach is recommended for people of all ages, and modifications can be made easily if health issues such as allergies, gastrointestinal disorders, dental problems, infections, and weight concerns, among others, arise. We discuss such issues in the chapters that follow.

5

Gastrointestinal Problems

Heartburn. Bloating. Gas. Diarrhea. Constipation. Alternating diarrhea and constipation. Abdominal pain. Are these symptoms haunting you? You're not alone. Tens of millions of Americans occasionally or frequently suffer with these symptoms, and tens of millions more experience them chronically. These problems can send you scrambling for relief, which the drug companies are only too happy to offer. Are you going to have Mexican food tonight? Better take a pill to help prevent heartburn. Do you experience bloating and gas after eating certain foods? There's a pill for you. Are you experiencing alternating diarrhea and constipation? No problem—just ask your doctor for a prescription.

Whether your child has diarrhea or you've been diagnosed with Crohn's disease or irritable bowel syndrome, or you just got back from a trip to South America and you brought home traveler's diarrhea along with your souvenirs, probiotics can help. And if you are a new mother and your infant is colicky, then this chapter may well be your favorite, because we will explain how to treat your child, and help you get some much-deserved relief as well!

Another important problem we tackle in this chapter is the use of medications for gastrointestinal distress. Twenty-five percent of adults in the United States take over-the-counter calcium-containing antacids, and millions more take prescription medications for GERD and other digestive symptoms. Despite the popularity of these medications, they all have side effects, and to make matters worse, these drugs often not only don't provide adequate relief, they also don't correct the cause of the symptom or disease. And the cause of these gastrointestinal problems, or at least a significant portion of it, can often be attributed to an imbalance of bacterial flora in your gut.

In this chapter we discuss the more common gastrointestinal symptoms and disorders and explore how probiotics and their helpers can provide you with the relief you need and deserve. First, however, we take a critical look at the medications that tens of millions of Americans take to combat gastrointestinal problems and how they damage the bacterial flora in the gut and thus jeopardize your health.

WHAT *NOT* TO TAKE FOR GI PROBLEMS . . . AND WHY

With tens of millions of people experiencing heartburn, indigestion, diarrhea, constipation, and a host of other gastrointestinal problems—many on a daily basis—it's not hard to understand why over-the-counter and prescription medications to treat these conditions is booming. Unfortunately, many of these medications not only don't solve these problems, they perpetuate and create new ones. (One example: In April 2007, production of Zelnorm [tegaserod], a prescription drug for irritable bowel syndrome, was suspended after the drug was found to cause an increased risk of myocardial infarction, stroke, and angina.) Here's the lowdown on some common gastrointestinal drugs.

Antacids

It's a very common practice for people to reach for an over-the-counter antacid whenever they experience heartburn, bloating, or gas, or even when they anticipate these symptoms. (You know the scenario: "We're having chili tonight. I'd better take an antacid before we eat or I'll pay for it later.") The trouble is, your health will pay later because you took the antacids.

Antacids contain one or more of the following active ingredients: calcium carbonate (yes, the kind you get in calcium supplements), aluminum salts, magnesium salts, and sodium bicarbonate. All of these substances neutralize stomach acids, albeit at different rates and causing different side effects. Aluminum salts dissolve slowly in the stomach and can cause constipation. Magnesium salts act more rapidly and can cause diarrhea.

Calcium carbonate is an inexpensive source of calcium and also the mainstay of antacid products (e.g., Tums, Caltrate, Oscal). It acts quickly and neutralizes stomach acids for a relatively long time. The ease of taking these supplements (they are available in chewable flavored forms) contributes to people overdosing on them, which can cause constipation and, with chronic use, much more serious medical conditions. Sodium bicarbonate (baking soda, or bicarbonate of soda) is the least expensive and most readily available of the antacids. As the soda neutralizes stomach acids, it releases carbon dioxide gas, which causes people to burp. In addition to disrupting the body's acid-base balance in the stomach and gut, sodium bicarbonate also (as its name implies) is a source of sodium, which may harm people who have high blood pressure or heart problems.

All the TV, magazine, and radio advertisements tell you that antacids are okay. You see commercials where waitresses serve antacids with the meal, as if chili or meatloaf with a chaser of calcium carbonate were perfectly normal parts of the diet.

But antacids are *not* okay. Antacids neutralize stomach acid, raising the pH level from very acidic—about 2—to between 3 and 4, which neutralizes about 99 percent of stomach acid. *When you neutralize stomach acid by taking antacids, you upset the natural balance of your intestinal tract.* Antacids are murder—literally—on probiotics and on your intestinal tract.

Stomach acid (hydrochloric acid) does more than digest food, it also acts as a bacterial barrier for the body. Every day you ingest food and other things that have microorganisms that have the potential to make you ill, or even cause death. According to the Centers for Disease Control and Prevention (CDC), food-borne diseases cause an estimated 76 million illnesses, 325,000 hospitalizations, and 5,000 deaths in the United States each year. (Many experts believe these figures are low, as many symptoms of food poisoning go unreported.) Experts have identified some of the culprits, including *Salmonella, Listeria, Escherichia coli* O157:H7, *Campylobacter jejuni,* and *Toxoplasma* as being responsible for many of the cases.

Stomach acid typically destroys these disease-causing substances before they make you sick. But when stomach acid is suppressed or neutralized, the protective barrier breaks down and the microorganisms get into the intestinal tract. If the environment in the intestinal tract is tipped in favor of lactic-acid-producing beneficial bacteria, the invaders will be destroyed. But if unfriendly bacteria have the upper hand, then you are highly susceptible to infection and illness, especially food-borne infections, which lead to food poisoning and the development of chronic degenerative disorders.

Proton Pump Inhibitors and Histamine-2 Blockers

The much-touted prescription drugs designed to dramatically reduce the amount of hydrochloric acid in your stomach are available in two categories: proton pump inhibitors and histamine-2 blockers. Both the inhibitors (e.g., Prilosec, Prevacid) and blockers (e.g., Zantac, Tagament, Pepcid) achieve this unfortunate goal by reducing the body's acid production rate. The lack of sufficient hydrochloric acid in the stomach leaves you vulnerable to the actions of bacteria that get into the stomach and then move into the intestinal tract. Again, if you do not have a sufficient amount of good bacteria in the gut you will get ill.

The damage does not stop there, however. Long-term use of proton pump inhibitors (longer than one year, which is not uncommon among users of these medications) is associated with an increased risk of hip fracture; in fact, an average 44 percent greater risk, ranging from 22 percent at one year to 59 percent at four years. Histamine-2 blockers also are associated with this risk, although to a lesser extent. The risk occurs because these medications reduce the ability of bone to absorb calcium. Both proton pump inhibitors and histamine-2 blockers also reduce the body's ability to absorb vitamin B12 and are associated with various side effects, including nausea, rash, headache, diarrhea, constipation, and abdominal pain.

The Probiotic Promise

While antacids and acid-suppression medications are some of the worst substances you can take to treat heartburn and other gastrointestinal symptoms, probiotics are the best. They are safe, effective, all natural, readily absorbed by the body, and easy to include in your diet or lifestyle. They are the logical choice for the gastrointestinal conditions that we discuss below.

As you read about the conditions and their associated probiotic programs in this and subsequent chapters, you will see two terms I will explain here: *flora blitz* and *flora sneak*. The flora blitz (which we nicknamed the "Shahani Blitz" when I and others were training with

Dr. Khem Shahani, one of the world's leading authorities on probiotics) is an approach in which you begin treatment by taking a high amount of probiotics for several days or longer, and then gradually reduce the amount over a period of days or weeks until you reach a maintenance level. The flora sneak takes the opposite approach: You start with a low amount of probiotics and gradually build up to the flora blitz, then reduce to a maintenance program. Most conditions respond best to the blitz; however, experience has shown us that the sneak works best in selected situations.

COMMON GASTROINTESTINAL DISORDERS

It's been said that it's more advantageous to have a strong gut than a good brain. Since there is such an intimate link between the cerebral brain and the second brain, you need to take steps to ensure and support the health of both your intestinal tract and your brain. That being said, in this chapter we look at the second brain in terms of its impact on gastrointestinal health. Although there are dozens of medical conditions that fall into the category of "gastrointestinal disorders," we focus on the more common ones that also respond best to treatment with probiotics and their helpers.

Gastroesophageal Reflux Disease

Acid reflux, also known as gastroesophageal reflux disease (GERD) or reflux esophagitis, is a chronic condition in which the hallmark symptom is heartburn, in which the liquid contents of the stomach reflux (regurgitate) into the esophagus. This reflux occurs when the sphincter (a ring of muscle at the bottom of the esophagus) malfunctions and relaxes between swallows. This malfunction then allows stomach liquids to rise up out of the stomach and into the esophagus. These liquids typically contain hydrochloric acid and pepsin (an enzyme), both of which are necessary to facilitate the digestion of food in the stomach. The refluxed liquid may also contain bile, which may get backed up into the stomach from the small intestine. The acid is believed to be the most damaging part of the refluxed fluids. Although the stomach has a lining that resists corrosion by the acid, the esophagus does not have this protective barrier, and so over time regurgitation can cause the lining of the esophagus to become inflamed and damaged, resulting in a condition called esophagitis (inflammation of the esophagus).

It's estimated that 10 percent of adults in the United States experience GERD symptoms daily, and one-third of Americans have symptoms at least once a month. Many people turn to one or more of the very popular antacids or antireflux drugs on the market that suppress the production of stomach acid. These drugs are absolutely the wrong treatment for GERD and related conditions for the reasons I discuss under "Why You Should Avoid Antacids." Once treatment begins, most people find that they need to continue taking medication. If they stop, their symptoms return, and there is often damage to the esophagus as well. These drugs have many side effects, but perhaps the most damaging is the one few people talk about: Chronic use of acid-suppressing medications creates an ideal environment for unfriendly bacteria and other pathogens to prosper and ultimately cause a wide array of health problems.

Checklist for GERD Symptoms

Persistent heartburn is the most common symptom of GERD. However, not everyone with GERD has heartburn. Heartburn is a burning pain in the center of the chest behind the breastbone. It typically begins in the upper abdomen and spreads up into the neck. Characteristics of heartburn may include:

__ Pain that can last up to two hours
__ Usually worse after eating
__ Usually worse if you lie down or bend over

Other symptoms of GERD may include:

__ Regurgitation of fluid from the stomach (and sometimes the small intestine) into the throat
__ Bitter taste in the mouth
__ Persistent dry cough
__ Tight feeling in the throat
__ Wheezing
__ Hoarseness, especially in the morning

In children, the most common symptoms are repeated vomiting, coughing, and other respiratory symptoms.

PROBIOTIC PROGRAM FOR GERD AND HEARTBURN

- Take 2.5 to 5.5 billion CFUs of at least five stabilized species with each meal until symptoms are under control.
- Reduce probiotic intake to the core plan level (see chapter 4) as your maintenance program.
- Take sodium chlorite ninety minutes before or after your probiotic dose—10 to 15 drops in 8 ounces of room temperature water or beverage. You can stop once symptoms disappear.
- Dietary recommendations: Reduce consumption of acid-forming foods (e.g., red meat, alcohol, caffeine, white sugar and other

refined products, spicy and fried foods) and include more alkaline foods, such as fresh vegetables and fruits, cottage cheese (no other cheeses), eggs, chicken breast, yogurt, tofu, and tempeh.

Irritable Bowel Syndrome

Irritable bowel syndrome is one of the most common, and often one of the most perplexing and annoying gastrointestinal conditions. Although this intestinal disorder is associated with signs and symptoms that can be severe (see "Checklist for IBS") and debilitating, the intestinal tract appears normal for many people who have the syndrome, which makes it difficult to diagnose. In fact, IBS can mimic more serious conditions, such as colon cancer, ulcerative colitis, Crohn's disease, and endometriosis.

According to the National Institute of Diabetes and Digestive and Kidney Diseases, about 20 percent of Americans, or up to 55 million people, suffer from irritable bowel syndrome. It affects three times as many women as men, and it develops before the age of thirty-five in about half of those affected. People who are diagnosed with IBS also often have an accompanying psychiatric disorder, such as hypochondrias or anxiety, which, although it does not cause the disease, does have a major impact on it.

Checklist for IBS Symptoms

Note: IBS is usually not diagnosed until abdominal pain or discomfort has lasted for at least three months and is accompanied by at least two of the following symptoms:

__ Distended abdomen
__ Alternating bouts of constipation and diarrhea

__ Abdominal and/or intestinal pain that is relieved by bowel movements
__ Mucous in the stools
__ Feeling of incomplete bowel movement

Also may experience the following:

__ Heartburn
__ Pain when swallowing
__ Fatigue
__ Urinary tract infections
__ Gynecological symptoms
__ Chest pain (not associated with the heart)

Fran's Story

Fran, a forty-two-year-old associate professor at a junior college, tells how she got relief using probiotics. "I was suffering with alternating episodes of diarrhea and constipation, along with bloating, gas, and abdominal pain, which made it real difficult at times to stand in front of a classroom. My doctor diagnosed irritable bowel syndrome.

"I didn't like the treatment options: antidepressants, antispasmodics—they were just temporary measures, they had side effects, and did nothing to really improve my health. So I changed my diet and included more fiber and fresh, organic foods, and that helped, and I made a conscious effort to reduce stress by practicing deep breathing exercises. But I still was experiencing frequent bouts of diarrhea and constipation, although they were much less severe, and gas was a chronic problem. I didn't want to take drugs.

"When I read about prebiotics and probiotics, it made sense. Even though I had improved my diet, I hadn't addressed the root of the problem, and these so-called 'good bacteria' seemed to be the answer. The most attractive part was that it's all natural, so I figured, why not give it a try. I bought prebiotic and probiotic supplements from a reliable company, took them with every meal, and within a few days I noticed an improvement in abdominal pain and gas. After a month, I couldn't believe the difference: No more on-again, off-again diarrhea and constipation, and the gas pains were virtually gone. As long as I take my supplements, I rarely experience any irritable bowel symptoms. And I don't think it's a coincidence that I have more energy and don't get colds like I used to."

PROBIOTIC PROGRAM FOR INFLAMMATORY BOWEL SYNDROME

- Flora blitz: Take 16.5 billion CFUs of five or more stabilized species per meal (three meals per day) for five days; then take
  - ✓ 11 billion CFUs per meal for five more days; then take
  - ✓ 5.5 billion CFUs per meal until your symptoms are under control.
- Stay at this level or reduce to the core plan level (according to your needs; see chapter 4) as your maintenance program.
- Recommended: Add a multienzyme supplement at each meal. Choose a supplement that contains a combination of protease, peptidase, amylase, and lipase enzymes. Begin to take the enzymes when you start the flora blitz and continue when you transition into your maintenance program.
- Dietary recommendations: Avoid refined carbohydrates, wheat,

corn, spicy foods, and popcorn; enjoy high-fiber foods such as fresh, organic fruits and vegetables, whole grains, and legumes.

Crohn's Disease

Crohn's disease (also called ileitis or enteritis) is a chronic, inflammatory disorder that can affect the entire digestive tract, although it most commonly impacts the lower part of the small intestine (called the ileum) and/or the first part of the large intestine. The inflammation is often painful and frequently causes diarrhea. Because the symptoms of Crohn's disease (see below) are similar to those of other intestinal disorders, including ulcerative colitis and irritable bowel syndrome, getting a definitive diagnosis can be difficult.

Although people of any age can get Crohn's disease, it is more often diagnosed in people between the ages of twenty and thirty. Its cause is uncertain, but the most popular theory is that the immune system launches an autoimmune response to certain bacteria, foods, and other substances in the intestinal tract and attacks them, which results in inflammation, the formation of ulcers, and other damage to the intestinal tract at all layers of the bowel. (This is unlike ulcerative colitis, in which the inflammation and ulcers form only in the top layer of the lining.)

The results of studies of the use of probiotics in the treatment of Crohn's disease have been mixed. The sole yeast probiotic (*Saccharomyces boulardii*), for example, can prevent relapse. In a group of thirty-two patients with Crohn's in remission, half were given mesalamine (an anti-inflammatory drug commonly used to treat inflammatory bowel disease) and half received mesalamine plus the probiotic. While six of the drug-only-treated patients relapsed, only one of the probiotic patients suffered a recurrence.

A combination of eight probiotics (*L. casei, L. plantarum, L. acidophilus, L. delbrueckii* subsp. *bulgaricus, B. longum, B. breve, B. infantis,* and *Streptococcus salivarius* subsp. *thermophilus*) was effective in significantly reducing the incidence of recurrence of Crohn's disease in patients who received the beneficial bacteria along with an antibiotic (rifaximin), when compared with the drug mesalazine alone. Thus far, however, not all studies of the use of probiotics in Crohn's disease have yielded positive results.

Checklist for Crohn's Disease Symptoms

__ Abdominal pain, typically in the lower righthand side of the abdomen, and often described as crampy or colicky. The abdomen may be swollen and sore when touched or light pressure is applied.

__ Diarrhea, which may contain blood, mucus, or pus. Episodes may occur as many as ten to twenty times per day and night.

__ Rectal bleeding, which can result in anemia if it persists.

__ Weight loss, usually associated with chronic diarrhea.

__ Loss of appetite.

__ Joint pain.

__ Fissures or abscesses around the anus.

__ Fever, which can be high in some people.

Other symptoms may include:

__ Mouth ulcers.

__ Skin ulcers.

__ Eye inflammation.

__ Rash.

PROBIOTIC PROGRAM FOR CROHN'S DISEASE
(FOR ADULTS AND CHILDREN AGE TEN AND OLDER)

- Flora sneak: For two days, take 1–2 billion CFUs of five or more stabilized species with breakfast only; then take
    - ✓ 1–2 billion CFUs with breakfast and lunch for two more days; then take
    - ✓ 2–4 billion CFUs with breakfast, 1-2 billion with lunch, and 1–2 billion with dinner for three days; then take
    - ✓ 2–4 billion CFUs with each meal for four days; then
- Begin the Flora blitz: take 16.5 billion CFUs per meal for five days; then take
    - ✓ 11 billion CFUs per meal for five more days; then take
    - ✓ 5.5 billion CFUs per meal until your symptoms are under control
- Stay at this level or reduce to the core program level (according to your needs) as your daily maintenance program.
- Recommended: Add a multipeptidase, enzyme supplement that contains a combination of protease, amylase, and lipase enzymes. Take the enzymes before each meal, starting at the beginning of the program and continuing after you transition to your maintenance program.
- Also recommended: 225 mg colostrum at each meal throughout the treatment program. You can stop once symptoms are under control.

PROGRAM FOR CHILDREN YOUNGER THAN 10 YEARS

NOTE: Capsules can be opened and the contents mixed with room-temperature food or beverage.

- Flora Sneak: 0.5 to 1 billion CFUs at breakfast and dinner for 2 days; then take
  - ✓ 1–2 billion at breakfast and dinner for two days; then take
  - ✓ 1–2 billion CFUs at each meal for three days; then take
  - ✓ 2–4 billion CFUs at each meal until symptoms are under control.

Colitis

Colitis, also known as ulcerative colitis, is a type of inflammatory bowel disease in which sores develop in the lining of the colon (large intestine) and rectum. The inflammation in the colon causes diarrhea, and the sores can bleed and produce pus. However, because the colon is long (average length, five feet) and divided into four main, rather distinct segments (ascending, traverse, descending, and sigmoid), different symptoms are characteristic of where in the colon and/or rectum the disease has settled (see "Checklist of Signs and Symptoms for Colitis"). Generally, symptoms are milder and the prognosis is better among patients whose inflammation is limited to the rectum and only a short portion of the colon.

Colitis can be a challenge to diagnose because its symptoms are similar to those of other intestinal disorders, especially Crohn's disease (see "Crohn's Disease"). Although colitis can occur in people of any age, it typically first appears between the ages of fifteen and thirty.

Several studies show that a combination of probiotics (*L. casei, L. plantarum, L. acidophilus, L. delbrueckii* subsp. *bulgaricus, B. longum, B. breve, B. infantis,* and *Streptococcus salivarius* subsp. *thermophilus*) can successfully treat mild to moderate colitis, serve as maintenance therapy for patients who are in remission, and improve the effectiveness of drug treatment (e.g., balsalazide or mesalazine, commonly used to treat colitis.

Checklist for Colitis Symptoms

Proctitis (limited to the rectum)

__ Mild, intermittent rectal bleeding may be the only symptom
__ Rectal pain
__ Sudden urges to defecate
__ Painful, unsuccessful urge to move one's bowels

Proctosigmoiditis (rectum and short segment of colon contiguous to the rectum [sigmoid colon])

__ Rectal bleeding
__ Sudden urges to defecate
__ Painful, unsuccessful urge to move one's bowels
__ May develop bloody diarrhea and cramps

Left-Sided Colitis (rectum, sigmoid colon, and descending colon)

__ Bloody diarrhea
__ Abdominal cramps
__ Weight loss
__ Left-sided abdominal pain

Pancolitis (inflammation that affects the rectum and entire colon)

__ Abdominal pain and cramps
__ Bloody diarrhea
__ Weight loss
__ Fatigue
__ Fever
__ Night sweats

A substance that contained both a probiotic and a prebiotic—a synbiotic—provided significant relief for people with ulcerative colitis in a study conducted in the United Kingdom. In the placebo-controlled double-blind study, patients with ulcerative colitis were given either a placebo or the synbiotic (*B. longum* and inulin) for thirty days. Once treatment was done, the investigators found that the treated patients had a significant reduction in chronic inflammation

PROBIOTIC PROGRAM FOR COLITIS

- Flora blitz: take 16.5 billion CFUs of five or more stabilized species per meal (three meals per day) for five days; then take
  - ✓ 11 billion CFUs per meal for five more days; then take
  - ✓ 5.5 billion CFUs per meal until your symptoms are under control.
- Stay at this level or reduce to the core program level (according to your needs) as your daily maintenance program.
- Recommended: Add a multienzyme supplement that contains a combination of protease, peptidase, amylase, and lipase enzymes. Take the supplement starting at the beginning of the blitz and continue after you transition to your maintenance program.
- Dietary recommendations: Avoid refined carbohydrates and spicy foods. Include high-fiber foods such as fresh, organic fruits and vegetables, whole grains, and legumes. If raw vegetables cause irritation, lightly steam them.

Leaky Gut Syndrome

Leaky gut syndrome is a very common gastrointestinal disorder in which the lining of the intestinal tract is much more porous (like a sieve) than normal. The gut is "leaky" because the unusually large spaces in the gut wall allow substances such as bacteria, parasites, fungi, partially digested proteins and fats, and waste to leak out of the gut and into the bloodstream. The large spaces allow larger than usual protein molecules to escape the gut before they are properly broken down. This causes the immune system to identify these molecules as invaders and produces antibodies against them.

These antibodies can cause a variety of problems, including food allergies and inflammation, which can result in conditions such as rheumatoid arthritis, chronic fatigue syndrome, colitis, or Crohn's disease (when the antibodies attack the gut lining), asthma, and vasculitis (inflammation of the blood vessels). Leaky gut syndrome also causes nutritional deficiencies, because the inflammation damages the proteins that normally carry minerals from the gut to the bloodstream. Therefore, people with leaky gut may experience deficiencies of magnesium (common in fibromyalgia), zinc (hair loss), copper (high blood cholesterol, osteoarthritis), and calcium (osteoporosis).

Checklist for Leaky Gut Syndrome Symptoms

__ Gastrointestinal cramping after meals
__ Bouts of diarrhea and constipation
__ Bloating and/or gas
__ General malaise
__ Food allergies
__ Muscle aches
__ Depression
__ Unbalanced gut flora

---

continued

Box continued

   __ Candida
   __ Fever

These symptoms tend to occur later in the course of the syndrome:

   __ Memory and/or concentration problems
   __ Headache
   __ Irritability
   __ Fatigue

PROBIOTIC PROGRAM FOR LEAKY GUT SYNDROME

- Start with 11 billion CFUs of five or more stabilized species per meal (three meals per day) and stay at this level until symptoms are under control.
- Include a multienzyme supplement at each meal. Choose a supplement that contains a combination of protease, peptidase, amylase, and lipase enzymes.
- Also recommended: Take 1,600 mg MSM, 20 mg manganese, and 2 million FCCPU bromelain at breakfast and again at dinner.
- Reduce probiotic dose to core program level once symptoms are under control.

Celiac Disease

Celiac disease is an autoimmune disorder in which people cannot tolerate gluten, a type of protein found in certain cereal grains, including wheat and related grains. In these individuals, the protein damages the mucosal surface of the small intestine and disrupts the absorption of nutrients.

The cause of celiac disease (also known as celiac sprue or gluten-sensitive enteropathy) is unknown, although an abnormality in the genes that are involved with the body's response to gluten protein appears to be involved. The disease affects about one out of 133 people in the United States.

Checklist for Celiac Disease Symptoms

Most common:

__ Abdominal cramps, distention, and/or bloating
__ Intestinal gas
__ Chronic diarrhea or constipation (or both)
__ Fatty stools
__ Weight loss despite a large appetite, or weight gain
__ Anemia, unexplained or due to a deficiency of folic acid, iron, B12, or all of these factors

Other symptoms:

__ Joint or bone pain
__ Fatigue and/or weakness
__ Depression
__ Defects in dental enamel
__ Osteoporosis, osteopenia
__ Infertility in men and women
__ Cold sores

PROBIOTIC PROGRAM FOR CELIAC DISEASE

- Begin with 4 to 11 billion CFUs of five or more stabilized species per meal (three meals per day) at each meal until symptoms are under control.
- Follow the core program.
- Strongly recommended: a multienzyme supplement at each meal, plus another dose between meals. Choose a supplement that contains a combination of protease, peptidase, amylase, and lipase enzymes.
- Dietary recommendations include avoidance of red meat and spicy foods, and including lots of fresh, organic fruits and vegetables, yogurt, rice bran, and black strap molasses.

Colic

"I don't know what happened," says Christine, a thirty-three-year-old first-time mother. "Daria was the perfect child for the first five weeks, and then she seemed to cry all the time. After a week, I was exhausted and so was she. She didn't seem to be sick, and her appetite was fine, so I was confused. My doctor said it was colic and that it would go away in a few months. A few months! My neighbor says she used to rock her baby for hours and drive her around in the car to get her to quiet down. I thought that would be my solution as well."

Fortunately, Christine contacted me and we started Daria on a probiotic program, and her symptoms virtually disappeared in a matter of days. This type of response is good news for mothers like Christine and for the up to 25 percent of all infants who experience colic. Although experts still are not clear as to what causes colic, the most common theories are that the speed at which food moves through the digestive system—either too fast or too slow—causes discomfort and thus the continuous crying, or that these infants have undiagnosed gastroesophageal reflux disease (GERD).

Checklist for Colic Symptoms

__ Excessive crying (more than three hours per day), in an otherwise healthy baby, that typically starts between the third and sixth week after birth and continues for about three to four months. The crying continues even though the infant is healthy otherwise; that is, he or she has the following characteristics:

__ Likes to be rocked, cuddled, and held. Unhealthy infants will not be consoled by these actions and will appear uncomfortable when handled.

__ Has a good appetite and a good sucking reflex. An ill infant will not.

__ Has normal stools or stools with greenish mucus. Diarrhea or bloody stools are not a sign of colic.

__ Spits up occasionally. Repeated vomiting and/or losing weight, however, are not typical of colic, and you should call your doctor if these symptoms occur.

__ Abdominal distention, along with gas or air in the intestinal tract.

__ Infant draws his/her legs to the chest in apparent pain and cramping and cries vigorously, often turning very red in the face and body.

PROBIOTIC PROGRAM FOR COLIC

- Mix the contents of one probiotic capsule (about 2 billion CFUs) containing at least five beneficial species with formula (or water if breast-feeding) and give at each feeding. Add just enough liquid to make a slurry, and then place it in the nipple of a bottle, enlarge the hole, and get your infant to suckle the slurry. Follow up immediately with a bottle (or breast-feeding).

- Also recommended is one multienzyme capsule (contents mixed with formula or water; choose a supplement that contains a combination of protease, peptidase, amylase, and lipase enzymes) with each feeding. You can mix the enzymes with the probiotics and thus eliminate a step.

- Once colicky symptoms disappear, continue to give your infant 500 million to 1 billion CFUs per meal as a maintenance program.

- Nursing mothers should take at least 4 billion CFUs per meal to help boost their immune system.

Diarrhea

Diarrhea is a very common illness that can affect people of any age and be short- or long-term, mild to severe. Approximately 100 million adults experience at least one episode of diarrhea per year, while children younger than three years of age typically have at least two events yearly. Diarrhea may be short-term, which is usually caused by a viral or bacterial infection; or long-term, which is typically associated with an intestinal disease or functional disorder (e.g., Crohn's disease, colitis).

Another frequent cause of diarrhea is the use of antibiotics, which is a special problem, because antibiotics kill both bad and good bacteria. The severity of the diarrhea often depends on the state of the intestinal flora: The more beneficial bacteria you have, the better your chance of avoiding diarrhea or of getting only a mild case. One double-blind, placebo-controlled study compared the use of a probiotic milk drink with a placebo for its effect on preventing antibiotic-associated diarrhea and found that the probiotic drink prevented 80 percent of antibiotic-associated diarrhea in hospitalized patients.

Sometimes antibiotics are prescribed to treat diarrhea, and when they are used to treat the intestinal disease caused by *Clostridium difficile,* chances are good the diarrhea will recur, if the intestinal flora is balanced in favor of unfriendly bacteria. Researchers have recently discovered that recurrence of the diarrhea can be avoided if patients are given the probiotic DDS-1 and/or *Saccharomyces boulardii* (available under the brand Florastor) along with traditional antibiotic therapy. In fact, this yeast-based probiotic was identified as the only probiotic effective against recurrence of diarrhea caused by *C. difficile.*

Checklist for Diarrhea Symptoms

__ Loose and/or watery stools
__ Abdominal pain
__ Cramping
__ Nausea and/or vomiting
__ Bloating

Symptoms associated with dehydration:

__ Thirst
__ Fatigue
__ Light-headedness
__ Dry skin
__ Infrequent urination

Constipation

According to the National Institute of Diabetes and Digestive and Kidney Diseases (NIDDK), constipation is defined as having a bowel movement fewer than three times per week and experiencing stools that are typically small in size, hard, dry, and difficult and/or painful to eliminate. Constipation is a symptom, not a disease, and is one of the most common gastrointestinal complaints, with more than 4 million Americans experiencing frequent constipation. Constipation occurs when the colon absorbs too much water, or if muscle contractions in the colon slow down and cause the stool to "stall" in the intestinal tract. The most common causes of constipation are poor diet (not enough fiber and/or liquids), stroke, and medication use (e.g., aluminum antacids, anticonvulsants, narcotics, diuretics, nonsteroidal anti-inflammatory drugs, ACE inhibitors, abuse of laxatives).

The Institute also notes that normal stool elimination varies by person, and that what is "normal" for some people may be only three bowel movements per week, while others may have one or more daily. I must take issue with this statement, and here's why:

Although moving your bowels just three or four times a week may be normal for many people, it is not healthful. Stool is waste; it contains toxic substances that need to be eliminated as soon as possible. The longer they linger in the colon, the more chance they can cause disease, including cancer.

Constipation itself is unhealthy. When you strain to eliminate stool, it places a great deal of stress on the colon. Over time, straining to defecate can cause thin sacs, called diverticula, to form in the colon walls. Food and toxic particles can collect in these sacs, become infected (a condition called diverticulitis), and eventually burst and release unfriendly bacteria into your body. Chronic straining can also cause the development of hemorrhoids or even rectal prolapse, in which part of the inside of the rectum protrudes through the anus.

Checklist for Constipation Symptoms

__ Abdominal pain
__ Bloating
__ Less frequent bowel movements
__ Dry, hard stool
__ Inability to pass stool
__ Straining to eliminate stool
__ Blood with stool
__ Rectal pressure or fullness
__ Rectal pain with bowel movement
__ Oozing liquid stool
__ Indigestion
__ Headache
__ Swollen rectal veins
__ Decreased appetite

Especially among the elderly, the following may be the only signs/symptoms:

__ Change in mental status (confusion)
__ Increased agitation
__ Incontinence
__ Unexplained falls
__ Low fever

PROBIOTIC PROGRAM FOR
CONSTIPATION AND DIARRHEA

- Flora blitz: Take 16.5 billion CFUs of five or more stabilized species per meal (three meals per day) for five days; then take
  - ✓ 11 billion CFUs per meal for five more days; then take
  - ✓ 5.5 billion CFUs per meal until your symptoms are under control.
- Stay at this level or reduce to the core program level (according to your needs; see chapter 4) as your maintenance program.
- Recommended: Add a multienzyme supplement at each meal. Choose a supplement that contains a combination of protease, peptidase, amylase, and lipase enzymes. Begin the enzymes when you start the blitz and continue throughout your maintenance program.
- Also recommended: sodium chlorite drops (10 to 15 drops in 8 ounces of water) three times per day, starting at the beginning of the program and stopping when symptoms are under control. Take ninety minutes before or after your probiotic dose.

Gastritis

Gastritis is an irritation, inflammation, or erosion of the stomach lining that can occur suddenly or develop slowly over time. It can be caused by a variety of factors, including chronic vomiting, stress, use of certain medications (e.g., aspirin, anti-inflammatory drugs), bacterial or viral infections, excessive alcohol use, or pernicious anemia. If left untreated, gastritis can cause a serious loss of blood or increase the risk of developing stomach cancer.

Checklist for Gastritis Symptoms

Note: Not everyone who has gastritis experiences symptoms.

__ Nausea or recurrent upset stomach
__ Gnawing or burning feeling in the stomach between meals
  or at night
__ Abdominal pain
__ Abdominal bloating
__ Vomiting
__ Indigestion
__ Hiccups
__ Loss of appetite
__ Vomit that contains blood or coffee-groundlike substances
__ Tarry, black stools

PROBIOTIC PROGRAM FOR GASTRITIS/INDIGESTION

- Flora blitz: Take 16.5 billion CFUs of five or more stabilized species per meal (three meals per day) for five days; then take
  ✓ 11 billion CFUs per meal until your symptoms are under control.
- Stay at this level or reduce to the core program level (see chapter 4) as your maintenance program.
- If you experience gastric symptoms between meals, take 5 to 11 billion CFUs when symptoms occur.
- Recommended: Add a multienzyme supplement at each meal. Choose a supplement that contains a combination of protease, peptidase, amylase, and lipase enzymes. Start to take the enzymes

at the beginning of the program and continue with your maintenance program. If the enzymes cause any gastric distress, discontinue them but keep taking the probiotics. Attempt to reintroduce the enzymes after about two weeks until you can tolerate them.

• Also recommended: sodium chlorite—10 to 15 drops in 8 ounces of water ninety minutes before or after your probiotic dose. You can stop taking sodium chlorite once your symptoms are under control.

BOTTOM LINE

Probiotics are proving to be highly successful in the treatment of a wide range of gastrointestinal diseases and symptoms. Compared with conventional prescription and over-the-counter medications used to treat such conditions, probiotics, along with enzymes and other bio-friendly substances, can help restore balance to the gut, and eliminate and prevent the recurrence, or significantly relieve the symptoms of, gastrointestinal disorders.

6

Allergies and Asthma

What would you do if there were an easy way to reduce by half the risk of developing allergic conditions such as eczema, hayfever, and asthma? What if you could give your child, or you yourself could take, a simple, safe supplement that would dramatically reduce or eliminate the symptoms associated with these health concerns? Forget the "what ifs," because you can: You can reduce your child's risk of developing asthma, atopic dermatitis, and other allergic conditions if you make sure he or she regularly gets a healthy dose of probiotics. You can fight the risk of developing allergies and asthma, or significantly improve your symptoms by restoring a healthy balance of friendly bacteria in your gut.

If you're reading this chapter, you (or a loved one) are probably suffering with an allergic condition or asthma that is causing you problems or discomfort in your life. The promising news is that exciting recent research shows that probiotics and prebiotics are effective against these often chronic and even life-threatening conditions. That means relief, elimination, and prevention of allergic conditions and asthma are possible with the help of selected microorganisms in supplements and/or foods. Here's the story. . . .

ALLERGIES AND ASTHMA TODAY: NOTHING TO SNEEZE AT

The word from the CDC and the American Academy of Allergy, Asthma, and Immunology (AAAAI) is not good: The incidence and prevalence of asthma and allergy diseases is increasing, especially among young people. Today, tens of millions of infants, children, and adults suffer with any one or more of the dozens of diseases and conditions that are associated with a hypersensitive immune system. For example:

- More than 50 million Americans have an allergy disease.
- Approximately 36 million Americans have seasonal hay fever.
- Approximately 20 million Americans, including more than 9 million children younger than eighteen years of age, have asthma.
- Chronic sinusitis affects nearly 35 million Americans.
- Allergic dermatitis (itchy rash) is the most common skin problem among children younger than eleven years of age.
- Atopic dermatitis (eczema) is one of the most common skin diseases, affecting between 9 and 30 percent of Americans. It is especially common among infants and children.
- Food allergy affects 6 to 8 percent of children younger than five years of age and 4 percent of adults.
- Approximately 30 million American adults have lactose intolerance.

WHAT ARE ALLERGIES?

"Allergy" is a general term for any condition in which individuals who have an oversensitized immune system react negatively to substances (allergens) that are generally harmless and in most people do not cause an immune reaction. Allergens can include bacteria, viruses, pollen, mold, medications, foods, dander, dust—literally thousands of substances can trigger an allergic response.

Generally, here's how allergies work: Let's say your immune system is overly sensitive to shrimp, but you don't know it. You go to a seafood restaurant with your friends and you try shrimp scampi for the first time. You enjoy your dinner, but unbeknown to you, the shrimp has triggered your immune system to recognize the food as an allergen, and your system stores away the information. In a few weeks, your friends say, "Hey, let's go to that seafood restaurant again," and you agree. This time you decide to try a shrimp cocktail, but this time you experience nausea, abdominal cramps, and a sudden rash. You've had an immune reaction. What happened?

The nature of an allergic response depends on various factors, such as the type of allergen, your level of sensitivity to the allergen, amount of allergen exposure, and the state of your immune system. Once an allergen enters or makes physical contact with your body, it triggers the production of antibodies, which in turn attach themselves to cells that contain histamine and other chemicals. These cells cause allergic symptoms when stimulated by antigens.

The type of symptoms you can experience is dictated by the part of the body influenced by the allergen. Thus, if you are sensitive to mold and you inhale mold spores, you may experience wheezing, nasal congestion, and a sore throat. If your skin reacts negatively to nickel and you put on a bracelet that contains the metal, you may experience a rash or hives. If shrimp is your downfall, you may experience tightness in your throat, difficulty breathing, or vomiting. In rare cases, people experience anaphylaxis, a life-threatening reaction to allergens. To help you identify different types of allergies and allergy associated conditions, see the explanations and checklists for each condition. *NOTE: The recommended probiotic program for asthma and allergy diseases is provided at the end of the chapter.*

Allergic Rhinitis

Dust, pet dander, pollen, molds, and other airborne substances that trigger a hypersensitive response, primarily affecting the nose and eyes, is known as allergic rhinitis. When symptoms are caused by pollen, the allergic rhinitis is commonly called hayfever.

Checklist for Allergic Rhinitis Symptoms

__ Itchy throat
__ Itchy nose
__ Mucus production
__ Cough
__ Wheezing
__ Nasal congestion
__ Runny nose
__ Tearing, burning, and/or itchy eyes
__ Red and/or swollen eyes

"I dreaded the arrival of spring every year," says Leslie, a fifty-three-year-old restaurant owner in Boston. "My allergies would drive me crazy. I had a runny nose, tearing eyes, and itchy roof of my mouth. I was miserable every day for months. If it weren't for running my restaurant, which I love, I would have moved." Fortunately, one of her customers told her about probiotics, and Leslie said she figured she had nothing to lose. After just three weeks of an aggressive probiotic program, along with some enzymes, her symptoms were "150 percent better," she says. "I couldn't believe it. And there are no side effects from the probiotics, unlike the allergy drugs on the market. I'll be taking probiotics all the time from now on."

Food Allergy

A food allergy is a hyperreaction by the immune system to a specific food or group of foods that are ordinarily harmless to the vast majority of people. The reaction is caused by an allergic antibody called IgE (immunoglobulin E). Note that food allergy and food intolerance (see "Lactose Intolerance") are not the same, because the latter does not involve an abnormal reaction by the immune system. However, probiotics can help both conditions.

Foods most often associated with an allergic reaction include eggs, peanuts, tree nuts, wheat, soy, milk, and shellfish (e.g., clams, shrimp, mussels, crab). Food allergies are more likely to occur in people who have a family history of allergies, and it often takes only a very small amount of the offending food to cause symptoms.

Checklist for Food Allergy Symptoms

__ Nausea and/or vomiting
__ Hives, which may appear and then disappear suddenly
__ Eczema (itchy, scaly red skin; see below)
__ Abdominal pain

---

continued

Box continued

___ Abdominal and/or intestinal cramping
___ Diarrhea
___ In rare cases, life-threatening symptoms (e.g., difficulty breathing, swollen tongue and/or throat)

ASTHMA AND OTHER CONDITIONS ASSOCIATED WITH ALLERGIES

Asthma

Asthma is a disease in which inflammation of the airways restricts the flow of air into and out of the lungs. During an asthma attack, the lining of the airways swells and the muscles in the bronchial tree get tight.

Not everyone experiences asthma in the same way: For some, cough is the main symptom; for others, shortness of breath and/or wheezing is the main problem. Symptoms also may last only a few minutes, but may go on for as long as several days.

Asthma symptoms can be triggered by inhaled allergens (e.g., molds,

Checklist for Asthma Symptoms

___ Coughing
___ Chest tightness
___ Increased production of mucus
___ Shortness of breath
___ Wheezing
___ Any symptoms initiated by triggers mentioned above

pollens, dust, pet dander) or by exercise, cold air, air pollutants, stress, drug allergies, or food. Many people with asthma have a personal and/or family history of eczema, hay fever, or other allergies.

Eczema (Atopic Dermatitis)

Eczema (also known as atopic dermatitis) is a chronic skin condition that is most often seen in infants and which usually disappears by age three. When it occurs in adults, it is typically chronic or recurring. Eczema erupts when something triggers a hypersensitivity reaction (similar to an allergy) in the skin, causing chronic inflammation. People with eczema usually have a family history of allergic conditions such as asthma, eczema, and hay fever. Evidence strongly suggests that pregnant and nursing women who take probiotics during and after pregnancy reduce the risk of their children developing eczema.

Checklist for Eczema Symptoms

__ Red, itchy, scaly rash, most often affecting the face, knees, and elbows.
__ Thickened, leathery skin that develops from chronic irritation and scratching.
__ Eczema may ooze or sometimes look dry.
__ Symptoms that worsen with dryness, temperature changes, exposure to water, and/or stress.

Contact Dermatitis

If you've ever had poison ivy or poison sumac, you've experienced contact dermatitis. This inflammatory skin condition is caused by direct contact with an irritating or allergy-causing substance. People who have a history of allergies are at increased risk for contact dermatitis. The most common type of contact dermatitis results from contact with detergents, solvents, and other chemicals, in which the skin looks burned.

The second most common type of contact dermatitis is associated with physical exposure to a substance to which you have become allergic. Some culprits include poison ivy and other plants, medications (topical), nickel or other metals (often in jewelry), perfumes, cosmetics, rubber, and fabrics. It is not uncommon for people to be able to wear a particular piece of clothing or jewelry on several occasions and then develop a reaction to it after repeated use. Some substances cause a reaction only if they are on the skin *and* the skin is exposed to sunlight (e.g., perfume, insect repellant, sunscreen).

Checklist for Contact Dermatitis Symptoms

__ Itching of the skin that was exposed to the substance.
__ Redness or inflammation of the exposed skin.
__ Tenderness of the exposed skin.
__ Localized swelling.
__ Lesion or rash at the exposed site. Lesions may ooze, crust, or drain, as well as become scaly, raw, or thickened.

Lactose Intolerance

Lactose intolerance is an inability to digest lactose, a type of sugar found in milk and milk products. It is caused by a deficiency of lactase, an enzyme that breaks down lactose. It is a digestive problem and not an allergy or allergy-related condition. However, because it is often confused with cow's milk intolerance, which *is* an allergic reaction, and which causes symptoms similar to those of lactose intolerance, we have included it in this chapter.

Checklist for Lactose Intolerance Symptoms

Symptoms can range from mild to severe and can begin thirty minutes to two hours after ingesting lactose.

__ Nausea
__ Cramps
__ Bloating
__ Diarrhea
__ Gas

HOW PROBIOTICS RELIEVE ALLERGIES
AND ASSOCIATED CONDITIONS

Are you allergic to ragweed, wheat, dust mites, cat dander, or other organic substances? In fact, what you are *really* allergic to is the protein in these items. Here's how allergies (and allergens—substances that cause allergic reactions) work, and how probiotics can help fight them:

Let's say you're allergic to cat dander. When cats lick themselves, the saliva dries on their fur, flakes off, and then lands on objects and floats in the air. When you inhale the dander, which contains protein molecules, the molecules enter your nose. The body has an enzymatic system that is designed to digest cat dander and other allergens. If the system is operating properly, two main steps occur: Enzymes called proteases break down the protein molecules into peptides, and then secondary enzymes called peptidases digest the peptides and transform them into amino acids. Once the amino acids are formed, the risk of an allergic reaction disappears.

This two-step process is successful only if you have enough of the right kinds of enzymes, and that's where probiotics come in. Probiotics manufacture enzymes. If you have insufficient levels of enzymes and probiotics in your body, then your body has inadequate defenses against allergens and your enzymatic system cannot handle them. The result is an allergic reaction. The best way to safeguard against allergies and related conditions is to make sure you provide your body with an adequate amount of enzymes and probiotics, through your diet and/or supplements.

What the Studies Show

Probiotics such as *Lactobacillus plantarum, L. rhamnosus, L. casei,* and *L. bulgaricus* can help protect against some allergic disorders, and some of these probiotic strains can reduce the intestinal inflammation that accompanies certain food allergies, including a cow's milk allergy that affects some neonates. Breast-fed infants of mothers who were given *Lactobacillus GG* had significantly improved atopic dermatitis compared with infants who did not get this probiotic. A placebo-controlled study of infants at risk of developing atopy found that those who were given probiotics during the first six months of life were half as likely to contract atopic dermatitis after two years when compared with controls.

In a double-blind, long-term study, a mixture of probiotics (*Lactobacillus rhamnosus* GG, *L. rhamnosus* LC705, *Bifidobacterium breve* Bb99, and *Propionibacterium freudenreichii* ssp. *Shermanii* JS), or a placebo, was given to 1,223 pregnant women two to four weeks before delivery. Once the children were born, they, too, were given either a placebo or a probiotic mixture that also contained prebiotics for six months. The children who received the probiotic/prebiotic combination were significantly less likely to develop eczema: There was a 26 percent reduction in eczema and a 34 percent reduction in atopic eczema. Along with this study, others have shown that probiotics are effective in treating infants and children who already have the disease.

Prebiotics also appear to be very helpful in preventing eczema (atopic dermatitis). A double-blind, randomized, placebo-controlled study of the use of prebiotics in 259 infants at risk for atropy was done by investigators in Italy. During the first six months of life, half of the formula-fed infants were given prebiotics (galacto-oligosaccharides and fructooligosaccharides) and half received a placebo. The infants who received prebiotics had significantly greater numbers of *Bifidobacterium* species compared with the controls, and also a reduced incidence of atopic dermatitis.

More Than Skin Deep?

Experts have noted that skin problems, such as athlete's foot, and the composition of perspiration are affected by what's in your gut. Therefore when your bacterial flora is out of balance, your skin may give hints about what's lurking deep within your gut. This should come as no surprise, especially when you consider that both the skin and the intestinal tract are charged with eliminating waste and toxins from the body (the skin through perspiration, the intestinal tract through feces).

A PROBIOTIC PROGRAM FOR ASTHMA AND ALLERGY DISEASES

- Flora blitz: Take 16.5 billion CFUs of five or more stabilized species per meal (three meals per day) for five days; then take

- ✓ 11 billion CFUs per meal for five more days; then take
- ✓ 5.5 billion CFUs per meal until your symptoms are under control.
- Stay at this level or reduce to the core plan level (according to your needs; see chapter 4) as your maintenance program.
- Include a multienzyme supplement at each meal. Choose a supplement that contains a combination of protease, peptidase, amylase, and lipase enzymes.
- Also recommended: 2,400 mg MSM, 30 mg manganese, and 3 million FCCPU bromelain when you get up in the morning, at midafternoon, and before bedtime. You can discontinue these supplements once your symptoms have resolved.
- Include sodium chlorite, 10 to 15 drops in 8 ounces of water, three times a day, taken ninety minutes before or after your probiotic dose. You can discontinue this supplement once your symptoms have resolved.

BOTTOM LINE

Symptoms of asthma and allergy diseases typically hit hard and often, so you need to treat them the same way: Start with a flora blitz, some enzymes, and a few other probiotic helpers to boost the blitz. Then, as symptoms improve and disappear, gradually reduce the probiotic doses and stop the helpers except for the enzymes, which, in people who have allergies, are necessary to help prevent allergies and allergic reactions. Then gradually reduce the doses until you end up with a daily maintenance program for probiotics.

7

Reproductive and
Urinary Tract Infections

If you are a woman, you probably already know that, unlike men, you are highly susceptible to both urinary and reproductive tract infections, and that these conditions often recur. What you may not know is that the majority of these infections are preventable if you make a few simple lifestyle modifications and adopt some healthful habits. One of the most effective and health-supporting habits you can include in your life is daily intake of probiotics.

Shirley, a thirty-nine-year-old graphic artist, says she wishes she had known about probiotics years ago, when she got her first urinary tract infection (UTI) at age thirty-five. Like nearly everyone who develops a UTI and seeks medical help, she was prescribed an antibiotic by her physician, and after she took the medication for the prescribed ten days, her symptoms were gone. Three months later, Shirley developed another UTI, and once she completed yet another round of antibiotics, she got a yeast infection, which her doctor also treated with an antibiotic. And that's when the nightmare started, says Shirley.

"For the next two years, it seems like I always had either a UTI or a yeast infection," explains Shirley from behind her drafting table in her home office. "During that time, I took several different antibiotics and tried a special Candida diet to get rid of the yeast infections, but nothing seemed to work. Along with the infections I always felt fatigued. But mostly I was just sick of being sick most of the time. In a way I was fortunate, because I do a lot of freelance work, and at least I had the luxury of being able to work at home whenever I felt well enough."

When a friend told Shirley about probiotics, she was eager to try them, although her doctor told her that probiotics weren't "proven" to work for UTIs or yeast infections. "I told him I didn't think I had anything to lose, since the antibiotics obviously weren't working, and that I didn't think the probiotics could be any worse than the drugs." Shirley started with an aggressive treatment program of probiotics and some additional supplements (see "Probiotic Program for Urinary Tract Infections"), and within a week she was feeling 100 percent better. She continued with the probiotic program and then gradually adjusted her doses until she reached a maintenance plan, which she continues to follow. Sixteen months after she first took probiotics, Shirley still has not had a recurrent UTI or yeast infection.

Shirley's experience is just one of many in which probiotics have proven effective in preventing new and recurrent urinary tract infections and reducing the risk of developing conditions that affect the reproductive tract. In this chapter we look at the characteristics of these common, recurrent infections, and how probiotics and their helpers can eliminate or, at the very least, significantly reduce the risk of urinary or reproductive tract infections.

URINARY TRACT INFECTIONS

Urinary tract infections are the second most common type of infection in humans, and are the reason for more than 8 million doctor visits each year. More than 50 percent of women experience at least one UTI during their lifetime, and 20 to 40 percent of them will, like Shirley, get recurring infections. Men are much less likely to have a UTI, although the infection can be very serious when one does develop.

Checklist for Urinary Tract Infection Symptoms

__ Frequent urge to urinate.
__ Painful, burning sensation in the urethra or bladder when urinating.
__ Feeling "washed out" or shaky.
__ Uncomfortable pressure above the pubic bone (in women).
__ Sensation of fullness in the rectum (in men).
__ Only small amounts of urine are passed, even though the urge to urinate is strong.
__ Cloudy, milky, or reddish urine may occur.
__ Fever is *not* a characteristic of a UTI alone, but it does indicate that the infection has reached the kidneys. Other symptoms of a kidney infection include nausea, vomiting, and pain in the back or side, below the ribs.

In infants and children (symptoms differ from those in adults and may be overlooked):

__ Irritability.

---

continued

Box continued

> __ Unexplained fever that does not subside. This may be the only symptom in children.
> __ Loss of appetite.
> __ Incontinence or loose stools.
> __ Failure to thrive.

Recurrence of a urinary tract infection and the lingering pain, discomfort, and lifestyle disruptions that it brings prompts many women to seek safe, effective ways to prevent reinfection. Jody, a thirty-one-year-old jewelry store manager, was one such individual. She had been experiencing an average of one to two UTIs per year for the past four to five years, and her doctor had prescribed an antibiotic each time. Unfortunately, each of these treatments was usually followed by bouts of diarrhea and "just feeling lousy for weeks." When Jody developed an infection in December 2005, she decided to bypass the antibiotics and to follow up on some information she had read about probiotics. She consulted with me and I suggested a probiotic program (see "Probiotic Program for UTIs"), and that she continue with a maintenance plan once her symptoms stopped.

Eighteen months later, Jody reported that she was UTI-free. "Since December of 2005 I haven't had one UTI," she says. "By now, if I hadn't been using probiotics, I would have had at least two, probably three infections. I can't believe it. This is great. And I also feel like I have more energy, so that's a plus!"

Causes of UTIs

Urinary tract infections in women are typically caused by bacteria in the stool that make their way into the bladder via the ureter. One common way this transfer of bacteria takes place is through improper bathroom hygiene—that is, wiping from the back to the front after a bowel movement and thus introducing bad bacteria (usually *Escherichia coli)* to the urethra. (*Escherichia coli* live a dual life: They are beneficial when they live in your intestinal tract, but can cause infection if they invade your urinary tract.) One reason women tend to have UTIs more often than men is that the bacteria have a very short distance to travel, as the urethra is close to the rectum in women. The urethra in women is also shorter than it is in men, so bacteria have a shorter pathway to travel to reach the bladder.

Other risk factors for UTIs include sexual activity, having several and/or many different sexual partners, urinary incontinence, diabetes, pregnancy, and low estrogen levels (associated with postmenopause).

Yet another common cause of UTIs is waiting too long to urinate. If you have a habit of waiting long past the time you first feel you need to urinate, your bladder—which is a muscle—will stretch and eventually weaken. A weak bladder is often not able to empty completely with urination, and urine that remains in the bladder increases the risk of UTIs and bladder infections.

Calcium, UTIs, and Probiotics

In recent years, more and more conventional health-care professionals have come to realize and appreciate the holistic nature of the human body and the importance of treating the entire person rather than just symptoms, as if the individual were separate from his or her bodily functions. Yet the idea of holistic medicine is not new: Traditional

Chinese medicine and the Ayurvedic medicine model, both of which have roots that go back thousands of years, are examples of a holistic approach to health.

Which brings me to the relationship that exists between probiotics, urinary tract infections, and calcium. This relationship is important for you to understand, because it illustrates a critical yet little known interrelationship that can result in a positive difference in your health.

Urine is supposed to be slightly acidic, as this helps suppress any bad bacteria in the urinary tract. If your urine becomes too alkaline—that is, if the pH value is greater than 7.45 (a pH of 7.35 to 7.45 is considered healthy), you greatly increase your risk of developing a urinary tract infection. One reason why pH levels rise is that some people take either too many minerals or the wrong types. One common example is calcium carbonate, a popular dietary supplement, taken by millions of people, especially to help prevent bone loss and osteoporosis.

Unfortunately, the calcium in most calcium carbonate supplements cannot be used by the body because it has not been processed through a technique called molecular chelation. In molecular chelation, elemental calcium is specially bonded (chelated) to amino acids, as it is in nature. Calcium supplements that have not been processed properly do not deliver the mineral to the bone receptor sites. Instead, the calcium enters the stomach and gut, and then it is eliminated without contributing to bone density. If you ingest calcium carbonate that is not biologically available to the body, not only don't you get the benefits of calcium for your bones, it can cause your urine to become too alkaline, and you greatly increase your risk of developing a UTI.

A Problem with Calcium Supplements

Although I'm glad so many women (and men) are concerned enough about preventing bone loss that they faithfully take calcium supplements, I'm also worried that many of them are taking the wrong form of the supplement, and thus little or none of the calcium is being used by the body. Here's why:

If you plant a fruit-bearing tree in soil into which you have added powdered calcium carbonate, the tree will draw up the calcium, and through the wonders of photosynthesis, it will bind amino acids to the calcium. The fruit from the tree will contain calcium that the body can use: When you eat the fruit, the calcium goes to tissues that need the mineral (e.g., bones). These tissues have bone receptor sites, which accept the amino acids and elemental calcium that is delivered to them.

When you take a calcium supplement, you want the same thing to happen: You want elemental calcium to be accepted by your bone receptor sites. However, if you take a calcium carbonate supplement that is not chelated properly—if the elemental calcium is not properly bonded to amino acids—the calcium will neutralize the acids in your intestinal tract, destroy beneficial bacteria in your gut, and upset the natural balance there. The same is true of any calcium supplement that is not chelated properly, including coral calcium, calcium citrate, calcium gluconate, oyster shell, calcium lactate, or calcium maleate. Avoid these products. (See "What Not to Take for GI Problems" in chapter 5.)

Getting Help for Your UTI

A big step toward preventing urinary tract infections involves avoiding the risk factors; that is, you need to respond promptly to the need to urinate and to practice good hygiene and safe sex. An even broader preventive step, however, can be accomplished by improving the makeup of the bacteria in your stool. Therefore, if you take probiotic supplements and/or include probiotic foods in your diet every day to help achieve and maintain a healthy balance of bacteria in your gut, you can significantly reduce the risk of developing a UTI. At the same time, if you do get a UTI, you can follow a simple yet aggressive probiotic treatment plan that can eliminate it for you.

In fact, research shows that women who frequently (three or more times per week) consumed fermented milk products containing probiotics (e.g., yogurt, sour milk, cheese) had a lower incidence of UTI recurrence than women who consumed fresh milk products. The probiotics in the foods studied typically included *Lactobacillus acidophilus* and *Lactobacillus GG*.

The use of intravaginal suppositories, which introduces friendly bacteria directly into the vagina, is another way to treat a UTI with probiotics. In a recent study, participants used suppositories that contained the probiotic *Lactobacillus crispatus* GAI 98322, which resulted in a significant reduction in the recurrence of UTIs. Apparently this strain of *L. crispatus* is not the only one that is effective in treating and preventing UTIs. A University of Washington School of Medicine study found that *L. crispatus* strain CTV-05 has high "stickability"—meaning the bacteria adhere very well to the target cells, which in this case were vaginal cells—and thus appear to be very effective in preventing recurrent urinary tract infections. Other studies show *L. rhamnosus* GR-1, *L. reuteri* RC-14, and *L. casei shirota* also help prevent UTIs.

Another way to directly treat the vagina is to use a probiotic douche, which you can do easily at home (see "Probiotic Program for UTIs"). A probiotic douche recolonizes the vagina with beneficial bacteria and also brings the pH level back to a healthful balance.

As you can see, various probiotic strains can be effective in the prevention and treatment of urinary tract infections. That is why I recommend taking probiotic supplements that contain multiple, stabilized species and strains, so you can enjoy the most benefit from these friendly bacteria.

PROBIOTIC PROGRAM FOR UTIS

- Take 16.5 billion CFUs per meal (three meals per day) of as many different stabilized species as possible for five days (if possible, include *L. crispatus, L. rhamnosus,* and/or *L. reuteri* as part of the mix); then take
  - ✓ 11 billion CFUs per meal for five more days; then take
  - ✓ 5.5 billion CFUs per meal until your symptoms are under control.
- Remain on a maintenance dose (see chapter 4).
- Take two cranberry softgels (300 to 400 mg each softgel) twice per day until symptoms disappear.
- Take 10 to 15 drops of 5% sodium chlorite solution in 8 ounces of water three times per day, ninety minutes before or after your probiotic dose, until symptoms disappear.
- Use a probiotic douche. Simply mix the contents of a capsule of a multispecies probiotic in some mildly warm water and douche twice a day until the symptoms disappear. If possible, a probiotic that contains *L. crispatus* is recommended.
- Also recommended is a multienzyme supplement that contains a combination of protease, peptidase, amylase, and lipase enzymes. Take a supplement with breakfast and dinner throughout treatment. Once you are on a maintenance program (see chapter 4), continue taking the enzymes even if your diet contains lots of raw fruits and vegetables.

REPRODUCTIVE TRACT INFECTIONS

Reproductive tract infections (RTIs) are caused by bacteria, viruses, or fungi that invade and attack the genital tract in both men and women. Of the three types of RTIs—sexually transmitted, iatrogenic (caused by a medical procedure or medically related activity), and endogenous—the type we are concerned with are *endogenous* infections, which are caused by an overgrowth of microorganisms that are normally present in the vagina. Although men also experience reproductive tract infections, they are much more likely to develop those that are sexually transmitted (e.g., gonorrhea, syphilis, herpes). Because sexually transmitted forms of RTIs are not responsive to probiotics, we focus our discussion to the two most common endogenous RTIs found in women: bacterial vaginosis and candidiasis. These vaginal infections are especially common among women of childbearing age.

Bacterial Vaginosis

Bacterial vaginosis is a condition in which the normal, healthy balance of bacteria in the vagina is disrupted by an overgrowth of unfriendly bacteria. It appears that several different species of unfriendly bacteria band together in causing this disease. Bacterial vaginosis is the most common vaginal infection that affects women of childbearing age, and develops in up to 16 percent of pregnant women.

Despite the fact that bacterial vaginosis is very common, exactly how women develop this condition is not entirely clear. Activities that can upset the bacterial flora population in the vagina and thus increase women's chances of developing bacterial vaginosis include douching (not, however, douching that uses probiotics), using an intrauterine device (IUD), and having a new sex partner or multiple sex partners. Having bacterial vaginosis puts you at increased risk of developing pelvic inflammatory disease, if you were to undergo a surgical procedure such as an abortion or a hysterectomy, and you would also be more susceptible to sexually transmitted diseases such as gonorrhea or chlamydia. If you were pregnant and also had bacterial vaginosis, you would be at increased risk for complications of pregnancy.

Several signs help physicians identify a true case of bacterial vaginosis. One is the presence of *clue cells,* which are cells that are covered with bacteria. Another sign is a noticeable reduction in the number of lactobacilli, a good bacteria, in the vagina.

Checklist for Bacterial Vaginosis Symptoms

__ Abnormal white or gray vaginal discharge that has an unpleasant odor; some women describe the odor as fishlike.
__ Burning during urination.
__ Itching around the vagina.

Note: About half of women who have bacterial vaginosis have no symptoms.

Probiotics and Bacterial Vaginosis

It makes sense that if a low level of lactobacilli in the vagina is a sign of bacterial vaginosis, then increasing that level by taking probiotic *Lactobacillus* species would be a logical treatment. In fact, several studies support this idea. In a study performed at the University of Washington, Seattle, for example, data were collected from 232 women with bacterial vaginosis who received an intravaginal capsule that contained either *Lactobacillus crispatus* or a placebo. The capsules were given twice a day for three days per month for three months. Overall, the women were very satisfied with the relief provided by the probiotic. In a later study in which two different species of *Lactobacillus* were used (*L. rhamnosus* GR-1 and *L. reuteri* RC-14) and compared with a medication called metronidazole, 90 percent of the women treated with the probiotics were cured of bacterial vaginosis compared with less than 50 percent of those who received metronidazole.

Candidiasis

Just the mention of candidiasis makes many women squirm. Twenty-five-year-old Candice still shudders when she thinks about how she used to suffer with this intensely uncomfortable vaginal infection.

"I still remember the first time I got candidiasis," she says. "It was October and I was a sophomore in college. I couldn't go to class because the itching was so bad. I was treated with antibiotics, and the condition cleared up in about a week. Then I got it again in the spring, and then again that summer. I remember thinking that I couldn't keep going through this; it was disrupting my entire life. I did some research and read about probiotics, and it made a lot of sense. I started taking probiotics every day, and since that time, more than four years ago, I haven't had another yeast infection."

Candidiasis is a type of fungal infection caused by *Candida,* which is the scientific name for yeast. In most cases, *Candida albicans* is the culprit that causes the often extreme itching, although the less common *C. glabrata* may be involved as well.

Candida is always present in the body, and as long as the beneficial bacterial flora are thriving and the immune system defenses are operating well, the body is usually able to keep the fungus under control. But if you take antibiotics or certain other medications (e.g., anticancer drugs, birth control pills, corticosteroids), if your immune system is weakened by disease or illness (e.g., cancer, diabetes, AIDS, malnutrition), or if you are pregnant, *Candida* can reproduce and grow uncontrollably. One of the most common targets of this overgrowth of *Candida* is the vagina. Seventy-five percent of all women are likely to develop at least one *Candida* vaginal infection during their lifetimes, and up to 45 percent will have two or more such infections.

Of Cows, Cowboys, and a Candida Diet

Over the years, the analogy I use when I talk about candida involves cows and cowboys. Candida is like a herd of cows, and the beneficial bacteria are cowboys. The cowboys put up fences and corrals to contain and manage the cows. They have a symbiotic relationship with each other. If the cowboys decide to ride into town and they leave the cows alone, the cows break down the fences and go in search of food. In the case of candida, that food is glucose, which is the same food the brain and muscles need to survive. Therefore, when people say they are on a "candida diet" and that they are going to "starve out" the candida by avoiding all carbohydrates, I tell them this is not a sensible approach. If you eliminate carbohydrates from your diet, your body will begin to use up protein to make carbohydrates. The results: Energy level declines, brain function suffers (your brain needs glucose from carbohydrates to survive), muscles atrophy, and dehydration can occur. Simply put, your brain and your body need carbohydrates; just make sure you give them healthy ones.

The sensible way to deal with *Candida* and candidiasis is to avoid the worst carbohydrates (i.e., white sugar, white flour, and products made with these ingredients), focus on healthy complex carbohydrates (i.e., whole grains, fruits and vegetables, legumes, seeds, and nuts), and hire more cowboys; that is, blitz your system with probiotics (see the probiotic programs at the end of this chapter). Once you do, you will bring those cows back into line and restore health and order to your reproductive system.

Checklist for Candidiasis Symptoms

__ Vaginal itch and/or soreness.
__ A thick, white vaginal discharge that looks and feels like cottage cheese.
__ Redness of the vulva.
__ Burning sensation around the vaginal opening.
__ Discomfort or pain during sexual intercourse.
__ Burning sensation when urinating occurs in some women.
__ Chronic fatigue, especially after eating.
__ Craving for starches and sugar (yeast thrives on sugar/ glucose).
__ Feeling "drunk" after eating a meal that is high in carbohydrates.
__ Bloating or gassiness after eating.
__ Chronic fungal infections (e.g., athlete's foot, oral thrush).
__ Anal itching.
__ Depression.
__Although less common, other symptoms include night sweats, chest and joint pain, memory loss, blurry vision, headache, insomnia, sneezing fits, food allergies.
__ Males with genital candidiasis may experience an itchy rash on the penis and/or jock itch.

Beyond Candidiasis

The impact of a vaginal yeast infection can go beyond the reproductive tract and ultimately affect the gut. That's when the yeast can cause the intestinal tract to become inflamed and cause an increase in the permeability of the intestinal membrane, which results in the release of protein molecules, undigested food, and other substances into the bloodstream. Once these foreign substances begin to circulate throughout the body, they can trigger a variety of problems, including food allergies and other allergic reactions, recurrent infections, joint and/or muscle pain, hives, fatigue, insomnia, headache, mood swings, confusion, multichemical sensitivity, and anxiety.

Fortunately, probiotics can help both prevent and treat vaginal yeast infections. Although research is ongoing, here's some of what we know so far.

Probiotics and Candidiasis

Experts have been studying the use of probiotics for treatment of vaginal yeast infections since the 1990s. In one study, researchers found that *L. sporogenes* was effective when it was used vaginally. In another study, twenty-nine women were treated with either *L. rhamnosus* GR-1 and *L. fermentum* RC-14 or *L. rhamnosus* GG alone, and the combination treatment was better at consistently preventing growth of *Candida albicans* when compared with use of *L. rhamnosus* GG alone. Yet another species, *L. acidophilus,* has also been shown to successfully treat candidiasis.

One important bit of information that investigators have found is that it is important to use more than one species or strain of probiotic when addressing candidiasis. Researchers studied the impact of various *Lactobacillus* species and strains against the growth of both *Candida albicans* and *C. glabrata.* They found that *L. delbrueckii* strains worked the fastest and strongest against *C. albicans* and also produced the largest amount of hydrogen peroxide, a substance which, like lactic acid, kills unfriendly bacteria. At the same time, the investigators also discovered that *L. plantarum,* which does not produce hydrogen peroxide, became active after 24 hours. Thus, the use of these two species gives both immediate and delayed activity against *Candida albicans,* but neither one has an impact on *C. glabrata.*

PROBIOTIC PROGRAM FOR CANDIDIASIS AND BACTERIAL VAGINOSIS

- Take 16.5 billion CFUs of as many stabilized species (include at least one or more of the species mentioned above: *L. rhamnosus, L. fermentum, L. delbrueckii, L. plantarum*) as possible per meal (three meals per day) for five days; then take
  ✓ 11 billion CFUs per meal for five more days; then take
  ✓ 5.5 billion CFUs per meal until symptoms are under control.
- Remain on maintenance dose (see chapter 4).
- Also recommended is a vaginal douche done once or twice daily until symptoms disappear. To make the douche, dissolve about 2 billion CFUs of as many stabilized species as possible in 4 ounces of warm water. Choose a probiotic supplement that contains bacteria only; other ingredients such as ascorbic acid can irritate the vagina.
- Also recommended is 5% sodium chlorite solution in water: take 10 to 15 drops in 8 ounces of water ninety minutes before or after your probiotic dose. Discontinue the solution once your symptoms have disappeared.

- For candidiasis only: Also take 600 mg of kyolic (aged garlic extract) garlic supplement daily until all symptoms disappear.
- The so-called candida diet is not recommended, but you should avoid simple sugars and highly refined carbohydrates (white flour products, white rice, sugar). Continue to include complex carbohydrates—fresh (organic if possible) fruits and vegetables, whole grains and legumes, nuts and seeds—in your diet. This is a healthful approach for both candidiasis and bacterial vaginosis.

BOTTOM LINE

Probiotics and their helpers can provide much-needed relief and protection from all-too-common urinary tract and reproductive tract infections. The addition of these natural healers to your life can not only help ensure you won't be bothered by these infections, they can also restore balance to the bacterial flora in your gut and a state of well-being overall.

8

The Immune System

You have a bacterial infection and your doctor has just prescribed a course of antibiotics that both you and she hope will knock out all the bad bacteria, eliminate the infection, and have you back to your old self in about a week.

Don't be so sure. In fact, that antibiotic will be killing more than bad bacteria—it will kill the beneficial, disease-protecting bacteria in your gut as well. And that's *not* so good. When the balance of friendly versus unfriendly bacteria in the gut favors the bad guys, the amount of toxic substances normally produced by the unfriendly microbes can become overwhelming and have harmful effects on the immune system. Once your immune system is affected, your entire body can feel the impact, because when the unfriendly bacteria are in control, the immune system must struggle to function efficiently, and that's when illness results.

The goal, then, is to keep your immune system functioning at its best, and probiotics can play a critical role in achieving that goal. Naturally, we want everyone to have a healthy immune system that is capable of warding off infections and threats of cancer and other serious conditions. And for many otherwise healthy individuals, the probiotic program we outlined in chapter 4 is an excellent way to maintain overall health.

But certain groups of people need to pay extra special attention to how their immune system functions, and sometimes otherwise healthy people need to address specific immune system problems at various times in their lives. So if you are chronically ill (e.g., have chronic fatigue syndrome, diabetes, fibromyalgia, asthma or another respiratory condition, or heart disease), are undergoing surgery, are experiencing a bout of flu or the common cold, and/or if you are elderly, your immune system needs are greater than those of healthier individuals. A probiotics program to boost and enhance the immune system can help meet those needs.

YOU AND YOUR IMMUNE SYSTEM

A healthy immune system depends on two key components: a nutritious diet, and a digestive system that functions well enough to allow you to get the most from your diet. Even if you eat only organic foods and drink only purified water, all the benefits of your efforts may be wasted if your digestive system cannot adequately metabolize the food and process the nutrients that your body needs to operate every organ system in the body. Beneficial bacteria are a critical component in the final breakdown (metabolism) of food in the gut.

One consequence of the inability to metabolize your food properly is the development of nutritional deficiencies, which in and of themselves cause and contribute to a wide range of health problems, from anemia to osteoporosis. Another consequence is a weakened immune system, which makes you more susceptible to countless health problems, ranging from the common cold to cancer.

I have found that patients who understand the role that probiotics play in enhancing the immune system are very enthusiastic about using probiotics for themselves and their families. So here we will break the system down into two parts and explore each one separately. The two parts are cell-mediated (or cellular) immunity and humoral immunity. We will limit our discussion to only the most important points in this highly complex world of the immune system and how it affects your health.

Cell-Mediated Immunity

Cell-mediated immunity is one way in which the immune system responds to harmful bacteria, viruses, and other health-damaging substances (pathogens). The immune system's response involves the actions of specific types of immune system cells, discussed below, rather than antibodies, which is how humoral immunity functions (see "Humoral Immunity").

Cell-mediated immunity protects the body in various ways:

- It activates T lymphocytes (or T cells), which are a type of white blood cell that attacks and destroys foreign invaders, such as viruses, fungi, protozoans, harmful bacteria, and tumor antigens.
- It activates natural killer cells (a type of lymphocyte that fights viruses and tumors) and macrophages (large cells that engulf and digest cellular debris and disease-causing organisms [pathogens])
- It stimulates the secretion of cytokines, a type of protein that influences and enhances the immune system response by activating macrophages and natural killer cells. Cytokines are also very important in wound healing and in regulating inflammation, as in arthritis.

All of this information about cell-mediated immunity will become relevant further on in the chapter.

Humoral Immunity

Humoral immunity is an immune system response that is directed by antibodies, which are special proteins the body produces in response to antigens—foreign substances such as bacteria, viruses, pollen, or toxins produced by bacteria within the body itself. Antibodies are produced by B lymphocytes (B cells) and bind themselves to antigens on the surfaces of the invading bacteria or other substances, which is a sign for them to be destroyed. Humoral immunity is so-called because the substances involved are found in the humours, or body fluids.

Now let's look at how probiotics are involved in both types of immunity in fighting two of the most common health problems, the flu and the common cold.

PROBIOTICS, THE FLU, AND THE COMMON COLD

Probiotics make significant contributions to the function of the immune system on several levels. *Lactobacilli,* for example, enhance both cellular and humoral immunity, while beneficial lactic acid–producing bacteria stimulate many of the immune system cells. Studies show that *Lactobacillus* GG improves the body's response to vaccines, including those for rotavirus and typhoid.

But what about the ever ubiquitous common cold and flu? You may have heard the expression, "we can put a man on the Moon but we can't cure the common cold." Well, although we still can't cure a cold or the flu, probiotics can take a lot of the misery out of these viral infections, and without the side effects medications can cause. In a double-blind, randomized, controlled trial of nearly five hundred healthy adults, investigators looked at the impact of probiotics on viral respiratory tract infections (common cold, influenza) during two winter/ spring periods (for a total of eight months). All the participants took a vitamin/mineral supplement daily, but half of them also took a probiotic that contained *Lactobacillus* and *Bifidobacterium* species. The number of people who developed a cold was similar between the two groups, but the subjects who took probiotics were ill for significantly less time than those who didn't take the probiotics (an average of two days less), had less severe symptoms, and experienced large increases in T cells, which are the good immune system cells.

You may have heard about the prescription medications on the market that can reduce the length of time you have to suffer with flu symptoms. These medications (e.g., amantadine [Symmetrel] and rimantadine [Flumadine], which are effective against influenza A only; and oseltamivir [Tamiflu] and zananivir [Relenza], effective against both influenza A and B) can, like probiotics, reduce the length of time you experience flu symptoms by one to two days. None of these drugs, however, enhance T cells and the immune system, nor do they provide the additional benefits provided by probiotics, which, in a nutshell, include improved gastrointestinal health and overall well-being. These medications also can cause side effects and they come with several precautions.

Oseltamivir, for example, has not been useful in the treatment of the common cold or any other respiratory illness that is not caused by influenza, yet many people unnecessarily take this medication when they don't have a definite diagnosis of influenza A or B (see "Signs and Symptoms of Flu" and "Signs and Symptoms of the Common Cold"). Since oseltamivir must be taken within forty-eight hours of the onset of symptoms if it is going to be effective at all, patients don't have time to wait to see if it is appropriate, and so they take the drug, hoping it will work. Side effects associated with oseltamivir include nausea, vomiting, bronchitis, headache, dizziness, stomach pain, and diarrhea, and there have been reports from Japan that it can cause hallucinations, self-harm behavior, and delirium among children who use this drug. Use of amantadine and rimantadine can cause similar effects: nausea and vomiting, dizziness, nervousness, and an inability to sleep.

So which will it be? Do you want to take body-friendly probiotics that will not only prevent the common cold and flu but effectively fight viral infections should they occur? Or do you want to take a costly prescription that, if it works at all, will reduce your length of illness by the same amount of time as healthy probiotics, and which may cause nasty side effects?

Checklist for Flu Symptoms

Note: Symptoms typically come on suddenly and can last from one to two weeks.

__ Fever (up to 104°F), and can last between 3 to 8 days
__ Chills
__ Muscle aches and pains
__ Severe headache
__ Weakness and fatigue
__ Loss of appetite
__ Sweating
__ Cough
__ Sore throat
__ Chest pain

The influenza virus can cause severe complications in the elderly or in anyone whose immune system is weakened by illness or disease, and it can damage the respiratory tract, resulting in bacterial infections.

Checklist for Common Cold Symptoms

Note: Symptoms typically come on gradually and primarily affect the nose.

__ Sneezing
__ Nasal congestion
__ Runny nose
__ Sore, irritated throat (typically, this is the first symptom)
__ Cough
__ Muscle aches
__ Headache
__ Postnasal drip
__ Decreased appetite

PROBIOTICS PROGRAM FOR INFECTIONS

- Take 16.5 billion CFUs per meal (three meals per day) of as many different stabilized species as possible, including any or all of the five species mentioned in the "General Immune System Functioning" program (*Bifidobacterium longum, B. bifidum, Lactobacillus plantarum, L. casei,* and *L. acidophilus* DDS-1) for five days. Then take

  ✓ 11 billion CFUs per meal for five more days; then

  ✓ 5.5 billion CFUs per meal until your symptoms are under control.

- Remain on maintenance dose (see chapter 4).

- Also recommend taking systemic enzyme supplements containing 2,400 mg MSM, 30 mg manganese, and 3 million FCCPU bromelain plus proteases and peptidase on an empty stomach three times per day—before breakfast, at midafternoon, and at bedtime. This dose can be reduced by one-third once the infection has cleared.

- Also recommend colostrum, twice a day, 225 mg dose each time. You can discontinue colostrum once the infection has cleared.
- Also take 10 to 15 drops of 5% sodium chlorite solution in 8 ounces of water three times daily ninety minutes before or after your probiotic dose until the infection clears.

THE IMMUNE SYSTEM AND THE ELDERLY

The body goes through many changes with age, and one of the most important changes is a decline in how quickly and efficiently your immune system responds to bacteria and other disease-causing invaders. One factor that contributes to the poorer response of the immune system in the elderly is the fact that people older than sixty have approximately one-thousandfold *fewer* friendly bacteria in their gut than do their younger counterparts. Therefore, older adults have an especially urgent need to bring the balance of friendly bacteria to the positive side. (You can read more about probiotics and aging in chapter 10. Here we are focusing on the immune system in the elderly.)

The decline in immune system function and efficiency is accompanied by an increased susceptibility to infection and disease, including cancer. Although the entire immune system is affected by aging, the one area that seems to be especially influenced in a negative way is T cell immunity.

T cells, as we noted earlier, are a type of white blood cell that is key to the immune system and is at the core of the body's cellular immune function, which means its ability to respond to specific pathogens, or disease-causing substances. Therefore, a decline in T cell immune function causes people to become less able to fight off or prevent an infection than they were in the past. This is one reason why older adults are urged to get a flu vaccination each year: Their age-related decline in T cell immunity makes them more susceptible to getting this viral infection, and, if they get it, to having a more serious, life-threatening case.

So, when researchers in New Zealand gave probiotic supplements to elderly volunteers, they looked at the impact on T cells. The volunteers were given *Bifidobacterium lactis* HN019 during the study, and when the investigators looked at their blood they found increased amounts of total, helper, and activated T cells and NK (natural killer) cells. The researchers also studied another group of elderly volunteers and found that *Lactobacillus rhamnosus* helped lymphocyte activity, which is important for another reason.

Lymphocytes are cells that are produced by the lymph glands, and one of their functions is to aid in the production of antibodies, which fight infection. As people age, they continue to produce lymphocytes, but the cells are less active and less effective than those produced by younger adults. Therefore, the immune system response of older people is less vigorous, making them more susceptible to infection and disease. Another complication of aging is that elderly individuals, especially those older than seventy, are more likely to produce autoantibodies, which are substances that attack the body rather than the organisms that cause infection and disease. Autoantibodies are involved in conditions such as rheumatoid arthritis and atherosclerosis, which are common among older adults.

PROBIOTICS AND SURGERY

Surgical procedures, whether planned or emergency, pose certain risks both during and after the event. Michael, for example, was scheduled for a hernia operation, and while he was not apprehensive about the surgery itself, he wanted to make sure his recovery was uneventful and quick. "I knew that the operation was not especially risky, but I also knew that all surgical procedures are associated with a chance of infection and other complications, and I wanted to prevent those risks." Donna fractured her leg in an automobile accident and was anxious to recover. "It's July now, and I want to be ready for skiing this winter, so I can't afford any complications." Priscilla underwent a mastectomy and said she was ready to "fight with everything she had" to beat breast cancer and any complications from the surgery.

Each of these people fought off the risks of infection and complications by taking probiotics, either postsurgery (Donna and Priscilla) or both before and after (Michael). Indeed, anyone who has a surgical procedure, including dental surgery, should safeguard him or herself with probiotics, before surgery if possible, and certainly after.

To find out just how effective taking probiotics can be in preventing postsurgical infections and complications, researchers have studied various groups of surgery patients. In a University of Chicago hospitals study, experts reported that probiotics helped prevent complications associated with surgery for ulcerative colitis and Crohn's disease, which include pouchitis and relapse. Given that up to 70 percent of people who have Crohn's disease will undergo surgery during their lifetime and that relapse is common after surgery, it's important that everyone who has the disease considers taking probiotics both before and after their procedure.

Similarly, 81 patients with liver cancer who underwent surgery were given prebiotics and probiotics either postsurgery only, or both pre- and postsurgery. Only 12 percent of patients who received the supplements both before and after surgery had a postoperative infectious complication, compared with 30 percent of patients who took the supplements after surgery only.

These and other studies aside, I believe it's common sense to protect yourself against postoperative infections and complications by taking probiotics before and after any surgical procedure. What have you got to lose, except some bad bacteria!

PROBIOTIC PROGRAM FOR POSTSURGERY

- Take 16.5 billion CFUs per meal (three meals per day) of as many different stabilized species as possible, including any or all of the five species mentioned in the "General Immune System Functioning" program (*Bifidobacterium longum, B. bifidum, Lactobacillus plantarum, L. casei,* and *L. acidophilus* DDS-1) for two weeks. Then take
    - ✓ 11 billion CFUs per meal for an additional two weeks.
- Remain on a maintenance dose (see chapter 4).

PROBIOTICS AND CANCER

At its most basic level, cancer can be defined as abnormal, often uncontrollable cell growth. Such growth occurs for reasons experts are still striving to fully understand. Some of those reasons include viruses, the presence of mutations in the genes, and exposure to carcinogenic substances (e.g., secondhand smoke, pesticides, various industrial chemicals), which change the DNA and stimulate renegade cell growth.

The role of probiotics in cancer is the subject of investigation, and it is also a relatively new area of study. Thus far, most but not all of the research has been done in animals, and the findings have been promising, suggesting that beneficial bacteria are useful as a preventive measure.

For example, probiotics can be used to help detoxify carcinogens and strive to maintain a favorable balance of good versus bad bacteria in the gut. As we mentioned in previous chapters, unfriendly bacteria produce toxins that destroy healthy cells and friendly bacteria. This destructive activity can make it easier for cancer to take hold and prosper. One reason it's so important to keep replenishing the supply of friendly bacteria in the gut with probiotics is that bad bacteria keep reproducing and are always trying to swing the balance to their favor. Unfortunately, if you are exposed to environmental toxins and practice poor lifestyle habits, you reinforce and support the bad bacteria. Therefore, the ideal way to keep unfriendly bacteria in check is to reduce the impact of these negative factors—for example, eat a more nutritious diet, reduce emotional stress, avoid pollutants, stay away from chlorinated water—along with regularly providing the gut with probiotics. If, however, the unfriendly bacteria are allowed to prosper, they can increase the risk of gene mutation and thus cancerous growth.

Colorectal Cancer

One type of cancer that appears to be especially influenced by probiotics is, not surprisingly, colorectal cancer. Colorectal cancer is the second greatest cause of cancer death in the United States and Europe. In 2006, a group of researchers in Rome, Italy, reported on their review of more than thirty studies of the impact of probiotics on colorectal cancer. Although the vast majority of the studies had been performed in animals and in cell lines rather than in humans, the results overwhelmingly pointed to the potential anticancer activity of probiotics. Studies in humans are underway, but the results were not yet available as of this writing.

Results of the animal studies show that the rates of colon tumor formation were reduced in animals who were given *Lactobacillus* strains. In particular, animals who received *Lactobacillus* GG showed a reduction in the activity of specific bacterial enzymes that may play a role in promoting cancer in the large intestine. It also appears that prebiotics can help fight cancer as well, at least in rats. Rats with chemically induced tumors who were given a mixture of inulin and oligofructose, as well as those given these prebiotics along with *Lactobacilli rhamnosus* and *Bifidobacterium lactis* had significantly fewer tumors compared to the control group.

Bladder Cancer

Two studies explored the possibility of recurrence of superficial bladder cancer in patients after they underwent surgery for their disease. A total of more than 200 patients were evaluated in the two studies, and the overall finding was that an oral *Lactobacillus casei* supplement was effective in preventing recurrence of superficial bladder cancer when compared with a placebo.

Enzymes

Digestion or intestinal tract problems are common among people who have cancer, and in many cases the conditions make it difficult for individuals to get adequate nutrition from their food. One way to help remedy this situation is to take digestive enzyme supplements. These enzymes, taken with meals, can help the body derive essential nutrients from food. They do not, however, have a direct impact on tumors. A few other studies in animals and in humans suggest that enzymes can improve survival in cancer patients. In a study of patients with stage III multiple myeloma who were undergoing chemotherapy, for example, those who took an oral enzyme supplement along with drug therapy for more than six months survived an average of three years longer than those who did not take the enzymes.

REVVING UP YOUR IMMUNE SYSTEM

While the core probiotics program works well for many people who are otherwise healthy, some men and women, and children as well, want or need added protection for their immune system. Their reasons for wanting added security vary: Some want to be prepared for the flu-and-cold season, or they know they are entering a time of great stress (e.g., going through a divorce, change in jobs, death in the family, cramming for exams). One popular reason is taking a trip abroad, as many people are uncertain about the quality of water and food in other countries. For whatever reason you may have, here is a probiotic program that features several bacterial species shown to be helpful in enhancing the immune system. Use it in good health!

PROBIOTIC PROGRAM FOR GENERAL
IMMUNE SYSTEM FUNCTIONING

- Take 11 billion CFUs of probiotics that have been identified as being especially helpful for the immune system: *Bifidobacterium longum, B. bifidum, Lactobacillus plantarum, L. casei,* and *L. acidophilus* DDS-1 at each meal for three to four weeks.
- Reduce dose to 5.5 billion CFUs per meal as a maintenance dose (see chapter 4).

BOTTOM LINE

Your immune system is your great protector against common, everyday assaults to your health, as well as more serious or catastrophic events. An easy-to-follow probiotics program can help support and enhance that defense system for you. Whether you want to plan ahead and help prevent postsurgical complications, boost your underlying immune system health, or put up barriers against the threat of the common cold, this chapter has a plan for you.

9

Weight Management

Could the "secret" of successful weight loss be beneficial bacteria? For many people, achieving and maintaining a balanced bacterial flora in the gut by consuming prebiotics and probiotics could be the answer to their weight-loss blues. This means that making probiotics and their helpers a part of your lifestyle could be *your* answer to weight loss and maintenance.

The first thing you need to do is banish the phrase "weight-loss diet" from your vocabulary. The most effective, lasting weight-loss diet is not a diet at all—it's a way of life. In this chapter, we discuss how the addition of probiotics and their helpers to a healthy eating program— one that is interesting, delicious, and easy to follow—can help you lose weight and keep it off. Part of the quest to lose weight also often involves lowering cholesterol levels, which is important for weight loss, a well-functioning heart, and overall health as well. Therefore, we also discuss the role of probiotics in reducing cholesterol levels and how this ties in with weight loss, eating habits, and fat metabolism.

HOW TO LOSE WEIGHT

When the topic of weight loss is raised, most people think of counting calories, calculating carbohydrates, eliminating sugar, reducing fat intake, and starting an exercise program—and all of these factors are important. Yet one obvious feature most people and health-care professionals overlook is an assessment of how well the digestive system is functioning.

Unless your digestive system is operating optimally, you cannot expect to reach and maintain your ideal body weight.

Think about that statement for a moment. If your digestive system isn't operating as it should—if you are not metabolizing your food properly, burning fat efficiently, deriving the nutrients you need from your food, and generating enough energy so you will feel like exercising—then your attempts to lose weight and keep it off will likely fail. That's because the digestive system plays a critical role in metabolism and energy production, two factors that are responsible for weight-loss and body-weight maintenance.

Monica, a forty-three-year-old mother of three, a part-time florist, and a self-proclaimed "full-time dieter," was skeptical about what she called "yet another diet scheme," but she knew she needed help.

"I've tried so many diets and diet plans, read so many diet books, that I should have made a career out of it," she says. "I'm an example of the classic story: I've lost the same twenty-five pounds many times, and it keeps coming back. One thing that doesn't keep coming back is my energy. I'm beginning to worry that all this yo-yo dieting is also damaging my health."

Monica has a right to be worried. Yo-yo dieting causes the body to reduce its metabolic rate, which means, although you *think* you'll lose weight by starving yourself or eating very few calories, the body recognizes the reduction in food input as starvation, and so tries to rescue you by reducing the rate at which it burns calories. Also, when you lose weight you lose both fat and muscle. Although muscle burns calories, fat does not. Therefore, when you stop dieting and begin to eat more normally again, your body will burn fewer calories than it did previously, because your metabolic rate is slower, and you will have less muscle to burn calories. Yo-yo dieting also increases your risk of coronary heart disease.

For Monica and millions of other people, the "secret" to weight loss and keeping it off is threefold: Take probiotics and their helpers on a daily basis; adopt a nutritious eating plan you can live with for life; and eliminate (or seriously curtail) factors that contribute to weight gain. We tell you all about the easy-to-follow probiotic program for weight loss and maintenance at the end of this chapter. But what about the factors associated with weight gain?

Cows, Antibiotics, and You

What do antibiotics and cows have to do with you and your quest to lose weight? Researchers in the agricultural arena have long known that giving antibiotics to livestock like cows and pigs results in significant weight gain. In fact, livestock owners routinely give low doses of antibiotics to their animals in their feed because the drugs change the animals' metabolism, improving their ability to retain fat and thus make them bigger, according to Gary Huffnagle, PhD, of the University of Michigan Health System. Naturally, fatter livestock means more profit for farmers, and so the use of antibiotics in livestock feed is a common and ongoing practice.

One reason that this is important is that *any* antibiotics you consume, either through a prescription ordered by your doctor or in the meat and dairy products that you eat, are very likely causing you to retain fat. This does not mean you should refuse to take any antibiotics that your doctor prescribes for you, but it does mean you should (1) talk to your doctor about any alternatives to antibiotic treatment any time he or she suggests them; and (2) take probiotics before, during, and after any course of antibiotic therapy, so you can protect your gut and facilitate fat metabolism (see chapter 8 on the immune system).

Although the amount of antibiotics and other harmful substances in an individual serving of meat, poultry, and dairy foods is typically low, the harm comes from the accumulation of these toxins in the body over time, with each meal you eat. Therefore, you should consider eliminating foods from your diet that contain antibiotics. If switching to a plant-based diet is too radical a change for you, you can turn instead to free-range, hormone- and antibiotic-free meat, poultry, and dairy products. These foods are becoming increasingly available in mainstream grocery stores and markets. Many people find that a combination of these two suggestions—eating more plant-based foods and only eating drug-free animal foods—is an easy compromise.

Weight Loss and Candida

"I just don't understand it," says Bridgett, a forty-three-year-old real estate agent. "I cut back on calories, I've been exercising three to four times a week, and I've lost a few pounds, but I can't seem to lose the bulge around my stomach. Even though I've lost weight, I still look terrible in a bathing suit!"

Gas, bloating, and abdominal discomfort are all too common among people who are trying to lose weight. Like Bridgett, they are partly successful, but the annoying and persistent presence of midsection fat, often accompanied by intense cravings for sugary foods, breads and pasta, and sometimes alcohol, is enough to make them give up and slide back to their old weight—and even add a few more pounds in the process.

If these symptoms have been part of your dieting and weight-loss experience, you have a lot of company. You also may be blaming yourself for not having enough "willpower" to fight off your food cravings. Yet the culprit for many people in this situation is the presence of an overgrowth of yeast, or candida. These opportunistic yeasts cause strong cravings for starchy and sugary foods. An overgrowth of candida, as we discussed in chapter 7, is very common today, given that so many people have a lifestyle that includes eating lots of sugar and ingesting antibiotics, both as medication and in food, as well as the use of birth control pills, cortisone drugs, and immunosuppressive drugs.

If you suspect candida may be contributing to your inability to lose weight and inches, review the information and probiotics program we discussed in chapter 7. Bridgett did, and she was pleasantly surprised. "No doctor had ever suggested that a yeast infection could be part of my problem with losing weight and all the bloating," she says. "After just a few weeks on probiotics and enzymes, I look and feel one hundred percent better. Now I'm shopping for a bathing suit!"

Getting the Most from Your Calories

Many people ask me if probiotics can help them lose weight, and then I explain how a well-functioning metabolism and digestive system are critical if they want to lose pounds and keep them off. In nearly every case, these people tell me that no one has ever told them about this important factor in weight loss, so they are grateful for the information.

Then I ask them this question: "Do you think you would lose

weight if you ate only one thousand calories a day?" They readily agree that they would, and mathematically it makes sense. One thousand calories daily is less than the average adult needs per day just to function minimally. Some clients tell me they have tried eating 1,000 calories, or even less, per day, and that they lost weight, but that they eventually gained all or most of it back.

But then I ask, "What would happen if you ate one thousand calories' worth of chocolate or candy every day? Would that be the same as eating one thousand calories' worth of vegetables and chicken? Would you lose weight if you ate the candy, or if you ate the vegetables and chicken?"

Here is a case in which a calorie is still a calorie, but how the body treats the chocolate calories and the vegetable/chicken calories is different. When the body doesn't get enough of the nutrients it needs to function properly—which would happen if you ate just chocolate or junk food—it fights back and goes into starvation mode. That means your metabolism slows down and calories are burned at a much slower rate as your body tries to conserve energy and fat.

However, if you were to eat 1,000 calories of vegetables and chicken, you would get lots of important nutrients and thus not trigger the body's starvation mechanism. You also would feel full and more satisfied, because you would be consuming much more food. Therefore, it's not just the number of calories you consume but also the nutritional content of those calories that count when you are trying to lose weight and keep it off.

Experts know, for example, that fat burns more slowly if you have low levels of vitamin B5 and protein, and that overall, the B-complex vitamins help convert carbohydrates into glucose, which is the fuel burned during metabolism. Probiotics are critical here, because they help manufacture B vitamins. Your body also needs protein, because it is used for the proper functioning of energy-producing enzymes that are responsible for burning fat. Therefore, if you eat too few calories, or if the calories you eat are largely empty of nutrients, you will not lose weight and you will harm your body.

To get the most from your food and lose weight at the same time, you need nutrient-dense foods and daily doses of probiotics to help you burn fat more efficiently. The combination of good food and probiotics will increase your energy level, which will improve your mood and help motivate you to enjoy daily exercise. Combine these benefits with the fact that probiotics also help eliminate renegade candida (and the cravings for carbohydrates that often accompany it) as we mentioned previously, and you have a recipe for successful weight loss and control. We offer you some delicious and easy recipes and menu ideas in chapter 12.

PROBIOTIC PROGRAM FOR WEIGHT LOSS

- Take 16.5 billion CFUs of as many stabilized species as possible per meal (three meals per day) for five days; then take
  ✓ 11 billion CFUs per meal for five more days; then take
  ✓ 5.5 billion CFUs per meal until you reach your goal weight.
- Remain on the maintenance dose (see chapter 4).
- Also recommended: taking a multienzyme supplement that contains a combination of protease, peptidase, amylase, and lipase enzymes. Take the enzymes with each meal throughout the treatment program. Once you are on a maintenance program (see chapter 4), continue taking the enzymes, even if your diet contains lots of raw fruits and vegetables.
- Incorporate more prebiotic and probiotic foods into your menus. See chapter 12 for recipes and tips.

CHOLESTEROL

One of the "perks" of taking probiotics to help you lose weight and keep it off is that these beneficial bacteria help normalize fat metabolism. When you normalize how your body processes fat, you reduce your risk of accumulating excess fat and plaque—including cholesterol—in your arteries, and you also help your body use that fat for healthful purposes, such as hormone production, brain functioning, energy production, and skin repair.

Some exciting new research shows that probiotics have the ability to break down cholesterol and use it for their own metabolism, which means there is less available to collect in your arteries. Studies in both animals and humans show that several strains of *Lactobacillus,* including *L.acidophilus* NCFM, *L. lactis* subspecies *lactis* strain N7, and *L. sporogenes,* have this ability and thus may prevent reabsorption of cholesterol back into the body's circulation.

(Note: *Lactobacillus sporogenes* was misidentified in the last century and reclassified as *Bacillus coagulans* in the late 1930s. Any references to *L. sporogenes* today may be an attempt to make it seem similar to *L. acidophilus* and other Lactobacilli. Although *B. coagulans* is a probiotic, it is a spore-forming bacterium and should not be confused with Lactobacilli.)

BOTTOM LINE

Dieting and weight loss remain among the main concerns of tens of millions of Americans, and it is a topic of conversation nearly everywhere you turn: talk shows, magazines, health clubs, billboards, and the Internet. Like so many health issues, multiple factors are involved: Most people don't lose a significant amount of weight and successfully keep it off by just eliminating cookies from their diet. Obviously, they need to do more.

The addition of probiotics and probiotic foods to a sensible, nutritious eating plan that you can live with, along with exercise, can make your weight-loss goal achievable as well as lasting. That's because when you have a healthy, balanced gut, your digestive tract, immune system, and metabolism are in synch and you better-utilize your food and nutrients, have more energy, and enjoy better health.

10

The Aging Challenge

With any luck, I'll be like a fine wine: I'll keep getting better as I get older," said Martin, a sixty-eight-year-old retired engineer and now part-time high school science tutor and oil painting enthusiast, "but to do that I need to avoid aging. I want to be a healthy old man." Martin has a positive attitude about growing older, and it is reflected both in his activities and in the choices he has made in his lifestyle. Along with his largely fresh foods diet, daily two-mile walk, and good sleep habits ("in bed by midnight and at least seven hours of sleep per night"), Martin takes probiotics every day at every meal. "I think of it as my insurance policy against getting old as I age," he says.

Martin is wise to take this simple but critically important step to protect his health as he grows older. He realizes that one of the problems with aging is that it is often insidious: Unless you have a medical condition that has drawn your attention to some specific deterioration or dysfunction in your body, you age silently—your cells, tissues, and organ systems quietly and gradually break down; hormone levels decline; metabolism slows and changes; and physical mobility and response become more limited. Naturally, the degree to which these and other aging features occur differs for each person, but the fact is that they do happen, and you *can* have an impact on how they happen.

Although you may think this chapter is only for "older" people, in reality it has something for everyone: Regardless of your chronological age at this very moment, you can benefit from the information in this chapter. Even though you may not be ready to adopt the probiotic program for aging that we provide in this chapter, our discussion will give you some insight into aging and how you or a loved one can advance in years without aging unnecessarily.

WHAT HAPPENS AS YOU AGE

Each and every day you have experiences, feel emotions, and encounter situations that you accumulate and store away in your memory bank. Good, bad, or indifferent, these memories are yours and will remain with you, to a varying extent, for the rest of your life.

Your physical body also accumulates "stuff" on a daily basis. The longer you are exposed to substances and conditions that contribute to physical aging and that destroy beneficial bacteria, the more your body will have difficulty restoring and maintaining a healthy environment in your gut, because it has accumulated substances that make reaching your goals more difficult.

The stuff we are talking about includes substances like chlorine from chlorinated water; preservatives found in processed foods; residuals from household cleaning products; carbolic acid from soft drinks; chemicals in secondhand smoke; food dyes; antibiotics from commercially raised meat, poultry, and dairy; and toxins in prescription and over-the-counter drugs. These are commonplace substances, so the first step in reducing or eliminating them in your life is to become acutely aware of them and then take steps to reduce their influence on the aging process.

"I used to drink soda nearly every day," says fifty-nine-year-old Marla, who recently started taking probiotics as a hedge against aging, "and then I learned that carbonated drinks contain carbolic acid, which upsets the pH balance and kills off good bacteria. I knew I had to stop drinking soda if I wanted to get the most out of the probiotics. It was a habit I found a little difficult to break at first, but I gradually made a switch to iced herbal tea and spring water with lemon and lime. Now I have a soda maybe once every few weeks, and to tell you the truth, I feel better: I have less gas and more energy, and I have the satisfaction of knowing that the probiotics I'm taking are giving me a chance to fight aging in a natural way."

Aging and the Gut

Among the age-related changes that occur throughout the body are those that affect the gastrointestinal tract. Recent studies show that the makeup of the bacterial flora changes with age. For example, the population of good bacteria such as *Lactobacilli* and *Bifidobacterium* species declines, the numbers of bad bacteria increase, and there's a reduction in the diversity of species. As we mentioned in chapter 8, people older than sixty have about one-thousandfold fewer beneficial bacteria in their intestinal tract than their younger counterparts. We also know that the mucosa of the gastrointestinal tract has the highest rate of cell turnover in the body. All of these facts make it much more likely that older people will develop constipation, irritable bowel syndrome, colitis, Crohn's disease, colon cancer, and other conditions that affect the gut.

Probiotics and their helpers can provide significant benefits for older adults, whether they want to help reduce the impacts of aging or treat symptoms and diseases that have already appeared. Olivia, a fifty-nine-year-old special education teacher, discovered the healing powers of probiotics for both herself and her eighty-two-year-old mother, who is a resident in a nursing home.

"I began to take probiotics and enzymes because I was having lots of trouble with irritable bowel," says Olivia. "I started with a high dose and gradually tapered down over the course of a few weeks, and now I'm on a maintenance program and feel great. And it occurred to me shortly after I started taking the probiotics that, if they were helping me they could help my mother too. She's confined to bed or a wheelchair, and quite often she suffers with constipation and gas, and she occasionally has urinary tract infections. I spoke to her doctor about giving her probiotics and enzymes, and he agreed. After just a few weeks, the change has been dramatic: Her constipation is virtually gone, and she has much better digestion with little or no gas. She has yet to get a urinary tract infection, so I'm betting that the probiotics are helping ward that off, too. The bottom line is, she's much more comfortable and her quality of life has improved because of the probiotics."

Aging and the Immune System

With advancing age, the ability of the immune system to respond vigorously to disease-causing substances declines. One of the reasons for this decline is that, with the passage of time, the body is no longer able to effectively assimilate and utilize the nutrients it needs to keep the immune system operating as well as it should. Another complication is that older people are more likely than younger people to have health and medical conditions that compromise their immune system and other organ systems, and more likely also to be taking multiple medications, many of which can have a devastating impact on the beneficial flora in the gut.

As the probability of an increase in the prevalence of disease among older adults looms on our doorstep, and as the aging population continues to grow, I find it encouraging that we are seeing more interest and studies on the impact of probiotics, prebiotics, and synbiotics, on intestinal and overall health, especially among older adults. This interest has led manufacturers to develop more functional foods and supplements, both of which can make it easier for older adults to get better nutrition and the probiotics and helpers they need to address the changing environment in their gut.

Enzyme Erosion

Probiotics have an intimate relationship with enzymes: Specifically, probiotics not only require enzymes in order to perform their many functions, they also manufacture enzymes. Therefore, probiotics and enzymes depend on each other; and so it is essential to find a probiotic with an enzyme delivery system. This would be a superior formula that would ensure an adequate level of both and help maintain those levels to stay healthy and fight the negative impact of aging.

An important point to know about enzymes is that, as you age, your enzyme system weakens through "food abuse"—that is, eating processed and cooked foods and foods loaded with artificial additives, all of which inhibit enzymes and their ability to perform. If, for example, you eat bread that contains an enzyme inhibitor (which commercial breads contain) and then you eat an apple (which contains enzymes), the chemicals in the bread will prevent the apple from digesting properly. The body always strives for balance, however, and so it will produce more digestive enzymes to make up for the ones that have been inhibited.

Unfortunately, you pay a price for this smart move by the body. Dr. Edward Howell, who is considered the father of enzyme research, explained the economics of enzyme production by likening the body's enzyme reserve to a bank account. You make deposits to your body's account whenever you eat raw foods, which supply enzymes and add to your reserve. This process also spares your organs from producing enzymes and gives them a rest. Whenever you eat processed foods, however, they lack enzymes, so you force your body to make withdrawals from your systemic enzyme bank account to produce digestive enzymes. You can exhaust your body's supply of systemic enzymes prematurely by diverting your organs from making systemic enzymes and having them produce digestive enzymes. If you continue to withdraw more than you deposit, which many people do, you will deplete your body of enzymes.

And you don't want to run out of enzymes, because you need them to live, and because probiotics need them to perform their tasks. To prevent overdrawing on your enzyme bank account, especially as you age, you need to (1) ensure you have an abundance of probiotics to help manufacture enzymes; and (2) make daily deposits into your enzyme account by eating raw foods and/or taking enzyme supplements.

Prebiotics and Aging

As you age, it becomes increasingly important to include fiber-rich foods in your diet to help maintain proper bowel function and to prevent constipation. Adults need 25 to 30 grams of fiber each day, and many if not most of those grams can be found in foods that are also prebiotics. That means you can get double the benefits when you eat prebiotic foods, which are good sources of soluble fiber that your body also needs.

Bifidobacterium species decline dramatically in older adults, and because we know that prebiotics can boost the populations of these essential bacteria, it's no surprise that the value of prebiotics in aging adults has been seen in several studies. In one, elderly men and women who consumed 8 grams of FOS daily experienced a significant increase in bifidobacteria, while another group of individuals saw an increase in these microorganisms when they ate 10 grams of soybean oligosaccharides daily. Malnutrition, calcium absorption, and lactose intolerance are also problems that often affect older adults, and prebiotics—as foods and/or supplements—can be helpful in preventing and treating these conditions.

Probiotics and Aging Skin

You already know that probiotics can be helpful for prevention and treatment of certain allergy conditions that affect the skin, including eczema and contact dermatitis. But is there any truth to claims that probiotics can help aging skin look younger or prevent skin from showing the classic signs of aging? Around the time this book was going to press, there were reports about probiotic serum products that claimed to make skin stronger and more resistant to aging. More specifically, producers of these products said the probiotic serum replaced the good bacteria to the skin that is lost with exposure to air pollution, sunlight, and stress. Can these claims be true?

Truthfully, I am not sure, but I hope to erase that uncertainty. That's why I am currently conducting my own investigations and am developing a natural probiotic facial treatment that will undergo rigorous testing to determine whether it can help aging skin.

PROBIOTICS PROGRAM FOR AGING

The probiotics program for aging involves taking higher doses of beneficial bacteria than what is used in the core program, because older people don't respond as quickly to dosing, and there's an age-related decline in the number of beneficial bacteria in their gut.

- Take at least 6 billion CFUs daily (2 billion at each meal) of five or more stabilized species/strains of beneficial bacteria (see chapter 4 for the list of stabilized bacteria).
- Include a probiotic food at each meal. This can be as simple as a few ounces of yogurt or kefir, or a side of fermented vegetables (see chapter 12).
- Include a prebiotic supplement or food with each meal. Detailed information on different prebiotic foods and supplements, as well as recipes and menu ideas, are found in chapter 12.
- Take a multienzyme supplement with each meal. Choose a supplement that contains a combination of protease, amylase, peptidase, and lipase enzymes.

BOTTOM LINE

You can't stop the natural aging process, but you can better ensure that your later years are as full of health and vitality as possible with the help of probiotics and complementary supplements. A simple daily probiotics program that also includes probiotic helpers can restore declining levels of critical, beneficial bacteria and enzymes to assist in keeping the gut, immune system, and other body systems in the best operating state possible.

11

Better Oral Health

If you stand in front of a mirror, open your mouth wide, and look inside, you'll see teeth, a tongue, and that funny hanging thing—the uvula. But what about what you *don't* see? The human mouth is a fertile breeding ground for bacteria, and your mouth is teeming with them. Similar to the bacteria flora in your gut, some of the bacteria in your mouth are friendly, while others are not. And like the bacteria in your gut, those in your mouth can have a significant and lasting impact on your overall health.

The use of probiotics for oral health is a relatively new area of research, and so studies are limited; but the findings thus far, including my own investigations and experience with patients, have been very promising. The newest findings join those of conventional wisdom: Your best defense against bad bacteria in your mouth and the problems they can cause is good oral health care, which includes daily brushing and flossing. You also want to maintain a healthy flow of saliva, which contains enzymes that destroy bacteria and viruses. These steps are important not only for your oral health, but for general health as well.

That's right: The health of your mouth doesn't stop there. Investigators have found that the bacteria in your mouth and inflammation of your gums are linked to other health problems in your body, including cardiovascular disease, diabetes, and osteoporosis.

These findings definitely make it even more critical to pursue and maintain good oral health. Thus in this chapter we take a close look at the role probiotics and their helpers can play in restoring oral health and in having a positive impact on overall health as well.

OPEN WIDE AND SAY "AHH"

Brush, floss, visit, clean. Most people are familiar with or have heard time and time again how to care for their teeth: Brush your teeth after every meal, floss at least once a day, visit your dentist once or twice a year, and make sure at least one of those visits includes teeth cleaning.

In reality, 36 percent of adults younger than sixty-five and 44 percent of those older than sixty-five did not visit their dentist within the last year, according to the National Center for Health Statistics (2006 report of 2004 figures), and nearly one quarter of those in the younger group have untreated cavities. Poor compliance with dental checkups and cleanings, along with a failure to brush and floss as recommended, are major reasons for yet another statistic: More than 50 percent of people aged thirty to ninety have gum disease, according to the U.S. Third National Health and Nutrition Examination Survey. In another study, which evaluated more than 500 patients aged twenty-five to seventy-three, investigators found that all of the participants had some degree of plaque, more than one-third of patients had plaque on more than 90 percent of their teeth surfaces, and more than 98 percent had bleeding gums. Clearly, dental disease is a problem that demands our attention.

Periodontal Disease

Periodontal (gum) disease is a general term for an infection of the tissues that surround and support the teeth. Among people older than thirty-five, periodontal disease is the main cause of tooth loss. Overall, however, most dentists say their patients are not adequately concerned about periodontal disease, according to an American Dental Association/Colgate survey, which explains the high percentage of people who have gum problems.

Periodontal disease is caused by the buildup of plaque, a sticky substance composed of bacteria that create toxins that damage the gums. In most cases, this buildup is the result of poor oral care habits: insufficient and/or improper brushing and flossing, and failure to get teeth cleaned professionally on a regular (yearly recommended) basis.

For more than 30 percent of the population with a European heritage, however, gum disease may have a genetic basis. According to the American Academy of Periodontology, these individuals may be six times more likely to develop periodontal disease, even though they practice good oral care habits. Therefore it is even more critical for everyone to take preventive steps to avoid gum disease.

Periodontal disease occurs in two forms: gingivitis and periodontitis. Let's look at each one separately.

Gingivitis

The early stage of periodontal disease, called *gingivitis*, is characterized by red, swollen, and bleeding gums. Unfortunately, gingivitis is often painless, and I say "unfortunately" because, if it were painful perhaps more people would take steps to treat it and stop it in its tracks. Many people either don't notice the signs or dismiss their symptoms as temporary or unimportant. The good news is that gingivitis is reversible and can be eliminated by daily brushing and flossing, and daily use of probiotics.

The effectiveness of probiotics against gingivitis has been documented in several studies. In one placebo-controlled, double-blind study conducted in Sweden, 59 patients who had moderate to severe gingivitis were given either one of two different *Lactobacillus reuteri* probiotic formulations each day, or a placebo. At the end of the fourteen-day study, the probiotic reduced gingivitis and plaque in 65 to 95 percent of the patients who took the supplement, but there was no significant change in the untreated (placebo) group.

If gingivitis is left untreated, it may progress to the much more severe gum disease called periodontitis (see "Periodontitis"). That's what nearly happened to Nadine, a fifty-one-year-old social worker who admitted that "I don't brush and floss as much as I should. I do casework and drive a lot, so I typically eat breakfast and lunch in my car while I'm driving. Unfortunately, I don't stop and brush, but I do swish with water when I can. And I chew sugarless gum."

Nadine also was not visiting her dental hygienist as much as she should, and she admitted that she had been urged by her dentist to brush and floss more regularly, as gingivitis was developing. Indeed, insufficient or improper brushing and flossing are the main cause of gingivitis. In some cases, use of certain drugs (e.g., phenytoin, calcium channel blockers, cyclosporine) can cause gum tissue to overgrow and lead to gingivitis as well.

"I began to notice that my gums would bleed sometimes when I brushed, and I didn't think too much about it until I started to feel tooth pain on my left side when I ate anything cold," said Nadine. "That's when I began to worry." Since most people with gingivitis don't experience pain, Nadine was lucky to get a warning and to heed it. She immediately adopted steps to change her bad habits: She now carries a toothbrush, toothpaste, and water with her at all times and takes the time to brush after eating.

"Sometimes I stop at a fast-food restaurant and use the restroom, sometimes I use the facilities in my office or at a rest stop. But I make sure I brush. I want to hold onto my teeth!"

Nadine also took two other preventive steps: She had a full-mouth disinfection, and she began to use probiotics (see "Full Mouth Disinfection"). Again, Nadine was fortunate because she learned just how important it is to follow a full-mouth disinfection procedure with probiotics, a winning combination that is effective not only for gingivitis, but for the more serious condition, periodontitis.

Periodontitis

For more than 5 million Americans per year, gingivitis advances to a more serious stage, called *periodontitis* (pyorrhea) which, according to the American Academy of Periodontology, is the main cause of tooth loss in older people. Although periodontitis is not reversible, it can be managed.

In cases of periodontitis, gum inflammation extends to the supporting structure of the teeth. The inflammation weakens the support and causes teeth to loosen and fall out. Most cases of periodontitis are the result of long-term accumulation of plaque in miniscule pockets that form between the teeth and gums. This plaque is the same substance that accumulates on heart valves, so if you have dental plaque, you also have cardiac plaque (see "Oral Health and Your Heart").

In the oxygen-free (anaerobic) pockets between your teeth and gums, bacteria thrive and reproduce unless they are treated. Symptoms of periodontitis include bleeding gums, swollen gums, bad breath, loose teeth or teeth that fall out, abscesses, and pain.

Checklist for Periodontal Disease Symptoms

__ Red, swollen gums.

__ Gums have "give" and are movable rather than being firm against the teeth.

__ Gums bleed easily, especially when eating, brushing, or flossing.

__ Gums that have pulled away from the teeth.

__ Development of abscesses or pus between teeth and gums.

__ Chronic bad breath.

__ Loose teeth.

__ A change in bite (how your teeth fit together when you chew or bite down).

__ A change in how partial dentures fit.

Oral Health and Your Heart

Periodontitis has been associated with an increased risk of coronary heart disease. What appears to happen is this: When the gums are inflamed and diseased, as they are in periodontitis and gingivitis, the bad bacteria can get into the bloodstream, either through cuts or other breaks in the gum tissue or mucus membranes in your mouth. Any type of dental procedure that could cause the gums or mouth to bleed, including routine teeth cleaning and even daily brushing and flossing at home if your gums bleed, also can allow bacteria to enter your bloodstream and affect your heart. Similarly, treatment to improve your oral health can result in an improvement in endothelial function.

Prior to April 2007, the American Heart Association (AHA) had recommended that patients who had certain heart conditions should take antibiotics before they underwent dental treatment, because it was believed that antibiotics would prevent infective endocarditis (bacterial endocarditis). However, the AHA's guidelines, published in *Circulation* in April 2007, state that most patients do not need to take antibiotics as a preventive measure before dental treatment. This decision was also endorsed by the American Dental Association, the Infectious Diseases Society of America, and the Pediatric Infectious Diseases Society, and here's why:

More and more research shows that the risks of taking antibiotics as a preventive measure outweigh the benefits for most patients. Those risks include adverse reactions to antibiotics (that can result in death for some patients) and the development of drug-resistant bacteria. For some people, however, preventive antibiotic treatment is still recommended. If any of the following situations are true for you, then preventive antibiotics are advised (along with probiotics): if you have artificial heart valves, a history of infective endocarditis, a heart transplant that has a heart valve problem, or specific congenital heart conditions. If you have any questions or concerns about the need to take antibiotics before a dental procedure, talk to your cardiologist.

Gum Disease and Other Health Problems

Some research has linked gum disease with premature birth and low-birth-weight infants. Pregnant women who have bad bacteria in their mouth may unknowingly pass along those pathogens to their fetus through the placenta or amniotic fluid and possibly cause premature birth. Oral health is important at all stages of life. Women who are planning on getting pregnant, however, should attend to their dental needs before becoming pregnant, because treating periodontal disease during pregnancy may be too late, as any infection may have already established itself in the mother-to-be and spread to the unborn child.

If you have diabetes, good oral health is very important, because the disease increases the risk of cavities, tooth loss, abscesses, dry mouth, and gingivitis. At the same time, poor oral health, and especially infections in the mouth, can make diabetes difficult to control, as infections can cause blood sugar levels to rise. Daily probiotics can help prevent such infections.

Full Mouth Disinfection

Full mouth disinfection (FMD) is a process in which dental hygienists perform tooth scaling and root planing to remove plaque above and below the gum line, plus the use of an antiseptic solution to irrigate the gums and clean the tongue and mouth. Many dentists use this procedure as both a preventive and treatment measure for gingivitis and periodontitis. Typically the procedure involves the use of chlorhexidine solution, but I have patented a natural procedure in which we use MSM, tea tree oil, and a cranberry gel to eliminate bacteria in the mouth. While this procedure is very effective, what makes my approach different from that of other full-mouth disinfection treatments is that I recommend that everyone follow an FMD with probiotics. *It is critical that beneficial bacteria be returned and restored to the oral cavity after full mouth disinfection.* And here's why:

Let's say you have a ten-square-foot spot in the middle of your lawn and you spray it with herbicides. What happens? The grass dies. So you rake up the grass and what remains is a bare spot where nothing is growing. After a few days, however, if you don't plant grass seed, weeds will begin to sprout up and soon take over the plot.

That's what happens in your mouth. After you undergo a full mouth disinfection (as many people do), your mouth is ripe for new growth. Bad bacteria is very opportunistic, and they are ready and willing to take over. That's why it's critical to bring in the probiotics after undergoing an FMD.

PROBIOTIC PROGRAM FOR ORAL HEALTH

Several specific bacteria have been identified as being especially helpful for the oral cavity: *Lactobacillus acidophilus* DDS-1, *L. plantarum, L. rhamnosus, L. salivarius,* and *Bifidobacterium longum.* These species are available in a tablet that people can chew and swallow daily after they brush their teeth and allow the residual from the tablet to stay in their mouth. This solution repopulates the mouth after it has been stripped of bacteria—good and bad—by full-mouth disinfection. Here is the recommended treatment following full-mouth disinfection:

- Each night after you brush your teeth, chew probiotic tablets that contain 6 billion CFUs of the abovenamed bacteria. Before you swallow the chewed tablets, swish the solution around in your mouth and do not rinse it out. Leaving the residual in your mouth allows the bacteria to attach and colonize.
- We also recommend you take an oral capsule that contains *Bifidobacterium bifidum, B. longum, L. casei, L. acidophilus* DDS-1, and *L. plantarum.* This combination is helpful in preventing the buildup of plaque in your mouth and on heart valves.
- As a general oral health preventive measure, you can open a probiotic capsule (preferably one that contains at least two of the abovenamed bacteria), place the contents on your wet toothbrush, and use daily.

You may be able to add a probiotic gum to your program against tooth decay. The German chemical company BASF has created a new strain of *Lactobacillus* called *L. anticaries,* which helps destroy the bacteria that causes tooth decay. The gum was scheduled to hit the market in 2007. According to results of company testing, the chewing gum can reduce the amount of bacteria in the mouth by fifty times. Other oral health products containing this probiotic, including toothpaste and mouthwash, may soon be available as well.

Oral Yeast Infections

The most common oral yeast infection is caused by *Candida*. The infection, called thrush, has traditionally most often affected infants and the elderly, but the increased use of broad-spectrum antibiotics, birth control pills, tricyclic antidepressants, and glucocorticosteroids, all of which can change the environment of the mouth, has led to a more widespread appearance of the infection among people of all ages.

Checklist for Thrush Symptoms

__ Yellow or smooth, creamy white coating on the tongue, palate, and/or inside of the cheeks which, when wiped off, reveals red tissue

Thrush is often asymptomatic. However, if symptoms do occur, they may include the following:

__ Burning or painful sensations in the mouth
__ Cravings for sugar, bread, or alcohol
__ Digestive problems
__ Fatigue
__ Depression
__ Joint or muscle pain

Should you say "cheese" if you have an oral yeast infection? According to a placebo-controlled, double-blind study of nearly 300 elderly people in Finland, patients with an oral *Candida* infection who ate cheese that contained probiotics had something to smile about. The four-month study showed that yeast levels were reduced by 75 percent in patients who ate the probiotic cheese, compared with patients who ate regular cheese.

Although eating cheese that contains beneficial bacteria may be a tasty and relatively effective way to eliminate bad bacteria in your mouth, I recommend a more potent, focused approach, as outlined below. I also encourage you to include probiotic foods at every meal.

PROBIOTIC PROGRAM FOR THRUSH

- Take 16.5 billion CFUs of as many stabilized species as possible per meal (three meals per day) for five days. Include the following species: *Lactobacillus acidophilus* DDS-1, *L. plantarum, L. rhamnosus, L. salivarius,* and *Bifidobacterium longum.* Then take
  ✓ 11 billion CFUs per meal for five more days; then take
  ✓ 5.5 billion CFUs per meal until symptoms are under control.
- Remain on maintenance dose (see chapter 4).
- Every night after you brush your teeth and before you go to bed, chew probiotic tablets that contain the abovementioned species. After you swallow the tablets, allow the residual from the tablets to remain in your mouth, as it helps restore good bacteria.
- Also recommended is 5% sodium chlorite solution in water: Take 10 to 15 drops in 8 ounces of water ninety minutes before or after your probiotic dose. Discontinue the solution once your symptoms have disappeared.
- Take a garlic supplement—600 mg of kyolic (aged garlic extract) garlic daily until all symptoms disappear.
- The so-called candida diet is not effective and therefore not

recommended, but you should avoid eating simple sugars and highly refined carbohydrates (white flour products, white rice, sugar). Continue to include complex carbohydrates—fresh (organic if possible) fruits and vegetables, whole grains and legumes, nuts and seeds—in your diet.

BOTTOM LINE

The mouth is the gateway of the gastrointestinal tract, a moist haven for bacteria, and, fortunately, receptive to doses of probiotics. Although research into the effectiveness of probiotics in oral health is not extensive, results thus far have been impressive, including those that show the advantages of introducing beneficial bacteria after full mouth disinfection to help reestablish a healthy environment in the mouth. Even the simple practice of brushing with powdered probiotics on your toothbrush each day is a great way to promote oral health.

12

How to Choose and Use

Probiotics and Their Helpers

You want to feel and look better. You want to protect yourself and your family (and your pets!) against illness and disease. You want more energy, better mood, and peace of mind. You've read about probiotics and their helpers and you believe they can help you achieve these goals.

So now you are standing in a nutrition store, or searching on the Internet, trying to determine which supplements to buy and which foods to include as part of your new prebiotic/probiotic eating plan. You have questions: Where should you start? Which form of probiotic, prebiotic, and enzyme supplements should you buy? How do you know which supplements deliver the doses that they claim on the label? Which prebiotic and probiotic foods should you include in your diet? This chapter is dedicated to answering these and other questions about how to purchase, use, and store prebiotic and probiotic supplements, and how to enjoy foods and beverages that contain and/or promote these beneficial ingredients.

PROBIOTICS: GETTING STARTED

We are going to make three assumptions here: that you have read the previous chapters; that you have little or no experience taking probiotics; and that you're ready to get started.

When you introduce probiotics into your gut, you want to make sure they enter an environment that is as friendly and nurturing as possible so they will thrive, reproduce, and do the job for which they were taken. Probiotic supplements and their helpers can provide significant health benefits, but *only if* you provide your body with a sufficient amount of quality, beneficial organisms as a foundation. Building that foundation is your first step. Then you can add to it and support it.

Planting a Probiotic "Garden"

For many years, probiotic experts and advocates believed that when it came to ingesting beneficial bacteria, you could treat your gut like a garden: If you provided it with good "seed" probiotics in one or two doses, they would colonize your intestinal tract and you could sit back and let Nature take its course. As the beneficial bacteria died off, you could "reseed" your garden with another dose, especially if your garden was poisoned with antibiotics, which would kill off the good bacteria.

Experts now know that that approach doesn't provide the protection you need. To continue with the garden analogy, the great numbers and aggressiveness of the "weeds"—bad bacteria—can be successfully overcome only if you first establish a sound foundation of beneficial bacteria, and then continue to feed it on a daily basis. That is why, in most cases, the recommended probiotic treatment approach to the various symptoms, ailments, and diseases discussed in previous chapters is the flora blitz. The large doses of probiotics used in the flora blitz allow you to establish a solid foundation in your gut, and you can support and enhance that foundation with prebiotics, enzymes, and other probiotic helpers, as noted in the various treatment programs.

How to Feed Your Probiotic Garden

Once the foundation is established, you can use a lesser dose of probiotics and support them with probiotic foods and probiotic helpers. Because probiotics are live organisms, they need to be nourished on a regular basis. The "right" conditions for beneficial bacteria to flourish include a warm, dark place, which the gut provides; but these organisms are also very sensitive to acidity (pH) levels. Therefore, the most significant impact on your gut environment comes from your food and supplement choices, because the microorganisms in your gut get their food from what you consume. Fortunately, you can control what your probiotics eat and thus whether your garden will thrive or wither. You can get the best results if you combine the easy guidelines that follow. Don't worry—in subsequent pages we provide you with plenty of tips and recipes to help you implement these suggestions.

- Take a high-quality probiotic supplement daily, preferably one with each meal. The minimum daily probiotic intake should be 2 billion CFUs and consist of as many different species and strains as possible. This is the recommendation for the core program (see chapter 4). Recommendations for other daily amounts associated with specific health problems are outlined in chapters 5 through 11.
- Make sure you get plenty of prebiotic foods in your diet: vegetables,

fruits, beans, legumes, whole grains, nuts, and seeds. Many foods in these categories are good sources of soluble fiber, and probiotics thrive on fiber.

- Include raw fruits, vegetables, and sprouted foods in your diet every day. Raw foods are a rich source of enzymes, which support probiotic health, and a good source of fiber as well.

- Include foods that contain polyphenols (e.g., artichokes, brussels sprouts, garlic, grapes, green tea, red wine, strawberries), which nurture friendly flora.

- Include fermented foods, such as yogurt, miso, tempeh, sauerkraut, or fermented vegetables in your daily diet, preferably at each meal. The active probiotic cultures in these foods help support the work of the beneficial bacteria in your gut. For example:

  ✓ Add a spoonful or two of yogurt to your breakfast cereal, such as oatmeal, farina, or whole-wheat flakes. When you do, you get both probiotics and prebiotics! However, yogurts do not contain a therapeutic dose of probiotics.

  ✓ Include pieces of tempeh in stir-fry or stews. If you have never had tempeh before, this is a good way to be introduced to this highly nutritious food. Tempeh is a fermented soybean food that has a consistency similar to meat and a nutty flavor.

  ✓ Enjoy fermented vegetables as a side dish instead of macaroni salad, cole slaw, or other common accompaniments to sandwiches and entrees.

- Avoid foods that contain refined sugars and animal fat. These foods feed and support unfriendly, disease-causing bacteria. When you eliminate these foods from your diet, you not only hinder development of bad bacteria, but also help stimulate the growth and production of beneficial bacteria.

- In addition to avoiding poor food choices, also eliminate activities and situations that can cause beneficial bacteria to die off. We talked about these factors in chapter 1, but just to refresh your memory, some of them include taking antibiotics, not getting adequate sleep, exposure to environmental toxins, and smoking.

HOW TO FIND QUALITY SUPPLEMENTS

As you may know, nutritional supplements are not regulated by the Food and Drug Administration in the same way that that organization regulates medications, so supplement manufacturers can sell their products even if they have little or no research to back up their advertising.

This does not mean you can't or shouldn't ask for evidence of any claims that a manufacturer makes. Reputable supplement manufacturers are happy to provide consumers with information about their products and any scientific evidence that supports their use. The Internet has made it easier to locate, investigate, and contact supplement manufacturers, as well as conduct research for articles and other information about probiotics, prebiotics, and enzymes.

Dolores is a thirty-eight-year-old mother of two who went in search of probiotic supplements when her doctor prescribed an antibiotic for a persistent bacterial infection. When she began to search on-line for the best supplement to buy, she was faced with dozens of different products from which to choose and became confused. First she researched to identify which beneficial microorganisms she should look for and learned that *L. acidophilus* DDS-1 and a variety of *Bifidobacterium* species would serve her best. Then she looked for an independent laboratory that could tell her how different supplements fared when they were tested, to make sure they contained viable amounts of the stated microorganisms. An Internet search lead her to ConsumerLab .com (see Appendix), a company that provides independent test results and information on nutritional and herbal supplements, so consumers and health-care professionals can make an informed decision when choosing such products. Armed with information, she felt more confi-dent about the purchases she made.

Choosing and Using Probiotic Supplements

Buy probiotic supplements that:

- have been manufactured properly and are not contaminated. Be-cause you can't witness the production of the products, you need to choose a reputable manufacturer. You can also check with an independent lab for viability.
- contain viable organisms. Some ways to help make sure you get viable bacteria is to choose species that have been stabilized (see the list in chapter 1), choose forms that are more stable (capsules and tablets are more stable than powders and liquids), and to al-ways use supplements by their expiration date.
- were stored, handled, and shipped properly. Refrigerated stor-age is usually recommended, but new technology has made it possible for some probiotics to retain their stability for two years on the shelf, unrefrigerated. However, refrigerating your probi-otics is a good practice, as it prevents unintended harm, such as exposure to sunlight or other light, or to heat sources, or to moisture.
- are sold in HDPE plastic or glass containers. Probiotics are anaer-obic, and may be damaged in the presence of oxygen.

Capsule, Tablet, Powder, or Liquid?

When it comes to probiotics, capsules are the preferred form of supplement for several reasons: They have a natural barrier against moisture, oxygen, and other contaminants; they are easy to use; they can be opened and the contents sprinkled on room-temperature food or in beverages, for easy consumption; there's no need to measure anything (unlike powders); and they travel well (liquids do not). Chewable tablets are the preferred choice for children and the elderly who have difficulty swallowing, and for people who are vegan (capsule coatings are often made from gelatin, which is an animal product).

Liquid probiotics do not remain viable for longer than a few weeks, and powders are constantly exposed to moisture and oxygen every time the container is opened. That's not to say that powders should be avoided completely, as they can be most helpful if capsules are not available and/or you need to make probiotic mixtures for children or to use in a douche. If you use powders, make sure the container is closed tightly and is stored in a cool, dry place.

How to Purchase and Use Prebiotic Supplements

Inulin and FOS supplements are available in tablets and powder. The average dose is 4 to 10 grams daily, which should be split into two or three doses rather than taken all at one time. Doses greater than 30 grams daily may cause gastrointestinal pain and discomfort, including bloating, diarrhea, and flatulence.

When purchasing inulin and FOS supplements, make sure the sources are chicory root (*Cichorium intybus*), burdock root (*Articum* spp.), and/or Jerusalem artichokes (*Helianthus tuberosus*). Here are a few other factors to consider when taking prebiotic supplements:

- Do not use prebiotic supplements if you are receiving whole-body radiation or radiation to the gastrointestinal tract.
- Prebiotic supplements may enhance the absorption of calcium and magnesium supplements if taken along with these minerals.
- Soluble fiber may reduce the effectiveness of other medications you may be taking, so consult with your doctor for guidance on when to take soluble fiber supplements.
- Pregnant and nursing mothers should use prebiotic supplements only if prescribed by their physician.
- Some lactulose preparations contain galactose, therefore do not take these preparations if you require a low galactose diet.

Synbiotics

Supplements that contain both probiotics and prebiotics are called synbiotics. This combination delivers a two-for-one advantage, as the ingredients synergistically enhance the actions of each other. In some cases, taking a synbiotic eliminates the need to take both a prebiotic and probiotic, if there are a sufficient number and potency of ingredients in the supplement. Synbiotics are available in capsule, chewable, and powder form.

How to Buy and Use Enzyme Supplements

Supplemental digestive enzymes are available in two basic categories: plant and/or microbial, and animal-derived. Plant-based enzymes are derived from several different sources, including pineapple, papaya, and mushroom-based fermentation. These enzymes perform very well in the gastrointestinal tract within a broad range of pH, temperature, and other environmental situations. One particular advantage of plant enzymes is that they work at the pH level present in the upper stomach. When you eat, food typically stays in the upper stomach for up to one hour before your gastric secretions kick in. During that hour, the enzymes in your saliva that started to digest your food continue to do so even when the food reaches your upper stomach. However, these salivary enzymes can digest only 10 percent of the fat, 30 percent of the protein, and 60 percent of the starch you eat, and they can continue to work only if your pH level is greater than 5.0.

Plant-based enzymes can function in a much wider range of pH: from 3.0 to 9.0. Therefore, if you take supplemental plant enzymes, they can begin to work immediately on the proteins, fats, and carbohydrates in your upper stomach, well before the stomach acid, hydrochloric acid, is secreted and neutralizes their activity.

Animal-based enzymes are derived from the pancreatic tissue of slaughtered cows and pigs. Supplements of animal-derived enzymes (e.g., pepsin, pancreatin, trypsin, chymotrypsin) have several disadvantages. One, they are effective only within a narrow pH range, and each enzyme is active only in specific sites. Two, animal-derived enzymes are destroyed by the low pH in the stomach unless they are enterically coated, but the coating prevents the supplement from dissolving and releasing the enzymes, which makes the supplement ineffective. Plant-based enzymes are superior because they can function throughout the digestive system.

PROBIOTICS, ENZYMES, AND PETS

Don't overlook your four-legged companions when shopping for probiotics and enzymes. Several companies have specially formulated probiotics, enzyme, and combination products for cats, dogs, and other animals. Many people consider their pets to be a part of the family and want to provide them with the best possible care. (Note: We focus on dogs and cats in our discussion, but products are available for other animals as well; see the appendix for suppliers.)

Like their human guardians, dogs and cats experience changes in their gastrointestinal tract that cause beneficial bacteria to die while bad bacteria proliferate, ultimately resulting in illness and disease. Conditions that cause such changes to the gut are typically stress-related and can include being left alone during the day, visits to the vet, thunderstorms, changes in diet, pregnancy, lactation, introduction of new household members (human and/or animal), moving to new location, transportation, and change in exercise.

Several circumstances are especially worth noting. One is your pet's food. If your pet were to choose its own food, you can be sure it would not include the dry kibble or cans of wet food you are buying now. The natural food for dogs and cats includes raw meat, which is rich in enzymes that animals need to help them metabolize their food properly. Most pet foods are processed to the point that natural enzymes are destroyed. Providing your pet with probiotics (which, as you'll recall, make enzymes) and enzymes is an excellent way to help them enjoy proper digestion and overall good health.

Pets that spend any time outdoors are often exposed to environmental toxins in the soil, air, and water. Dogs and cats enjoy digging and lying in the dirt, eating grass and other vegetation, and drinking water from puddles. Probiotics can help protect your pets from disease-causing microorganisms and other contaminants found in the environment. If you feed your pet a raw food diet, probiotic supplements are critical.

A serious problem that occurs with dogs and cats is that when they are ill, their gastrointestinal systems shut down and their nutrients are then targeted for the immune system. In most cases, these animals have only about 24 hours' worth of energy stored in their muscles, and when this supply is depleted, the body must burn fat for energy. If your dog or cat cannot recover from its illness before the energy supply runs out, he or she will die.

The use of probiotics can help your pet's health and well-being in several ways. Beneficial organisms can metabolize food that remains in the gastrointestinal tract even after the system shuts down, which means your pet can continue to get energy from the food until it runs out. This gives your pet more time to recuperate. Probiotics also boost the immune system and thus help it fight the infection or disease. Yet another advantage is that probiotics help prevent diarrhea, which can be deadly for pets, especially when they are already ill.

As they do in humans, antibiotics will kill beneficial microorganisms in your pet, opening the door for opportunistic infections. If your veterinarian prescribes antibiotics for your pet, make sure you begin probiotics at an accelerated rate and continue that rate for a week or two after the medication course is done. The probiotics will not only help prevent secondary infections but may help your pet recover faster as well.

PROBIOTICS PROGRAM FOR PETS

- Look for products that contain at least three or four species of beneficial bacteria, plus enzyme supplements that contain protease, lipase, amylase, and peptidase enzymes.
- For pets who are otherwise healthy but experience minimal stress and/or have minor digestive problems (e.g., gas, occasional diarrhea), give probiotics and enzymes once daily, according to label

directions. The amount depends on the weight of your pet or the amount of food consumed.

- For pets who experience chronic stress and/or who are ill, give concentrated probiotics supplements and enzymes twice daily, according to label directions, until symptoms disappear, then follow a once-a-day dosing. Concentrated formulas provide doses that are three or more times greater than regular dosing and are like the "flora blitz" we discussed in other chapters.

FOOD, GLORIOUS FOOD

When all is said and done, the best way to get your nutrients—probiotics, prebiotics, enzymes, vitamins, minerals, and other "good stuff"—is nature's way, in fresh food. When you choose wholesome, unrefined foods, you get nutrients in a form that is complete, synergistic, and natural to the body. Therefore, in all our discussions about food, we encourage you to purchase and use fresh, organic and/or free-range and hormone-free (when applicable) items that have been minimally refined/processed or completely unrefined/unprocessed whenever possible.

Probiotic Foods

Probiotic foods are foods that contain live beneficial bacteria, naturally and/or as an additive. Perhaps the most recognized probiotic foods are yogurt and acidophilus milk, the latter of which was first introduced in the 1920s as a probiotic food to help people who had problems digesting milk. It can now be found in conventional supermarkets, usually alongside regular milk products.

It has become increasingly common for food manufacturers to add beneficial bacteria, antioxidants, and other health-promoting substances to foods to "transform" those foods into "functional foods." When beneficial bacteria are added, the foods are sometimes referred to as "probiotics." In the case of foods like yogurt, the raw, unpasteurized product naturally contains lots of beneficial bacteria. This is the type of yogurt people used to eat in the past and that is still consumed by many people in Europe and other countries.

Yogurt Today

But many yogurts today, especially in the United States, undergo pasteurization, a process that kills bacteria. To transform such yogurts into "probiotics," many food manufacturers add beneficial bacteria back into their products after pasteurization. Always check the label of any yogurt products you buy to make sure they contain the words "contains live and active cultures." You should always check the expiration date on yogurt products, because the bacteria die over time. The bacteria most often added back are *S. thermophilus, Lactobacillus acidophilus, L. bulgaricus, L.* GG, and various *Bifidobacterium* species, although some manufacturers do not list individual species and/or strains of the bacteria they have used. Yogurt manufacturers also usually do not list the number of live cultures their products contain. You can contact individual yogurt makers by phone, e-mail, or regular mail, and ask for this information.

You can also look for the National Yogurt Association's Live & Active Cultures seal on your yogurt, which indicates that the product contained live cultures when it was made. This is still no guarantee, however, that the product was shipped, stored, or displayed in ways necessary to keep the beneficial bacteria alive and viable. As a general rule, avoid yogurts that contain preservatives, added sugar, and/or fruit.

An alternative to commercial yogurt is homemade yogurt. More and more people are finding that making their own yogurt is a healthy, fun, and less expensive way to supplement their probiotic "garden." See "Making Yogurt" in this chapter.

Kefir—The New Milk?

Kefir is a dairy product that is fermented with special grains that are a mixture of bacteria and yeasts. The yeasts produce carbon dioxide and alcohol, which give kefir both a distinct taste and make it fizzy.

Although kefir has been consumed for centuries by people in many different cultures and valued for its health benefits, science has only recently taken a serious look at those health claims. In a study at Ohio State University, Hertzler and Clancy set out to determine whether kefir improves lactose tolerance and digestion in adults who have lactose intolerance. Fifteen otherwise healthy adults participated in the study in which they had meals that contained 2% milk that contained lactose, plain and flavored kefir, and plain and flavored yogurt after an overnight fast.

The plain kefir, plain yogurt, and flavored yogurt provided the most dramatic results, significantly improving lactose digestion and tolerance. The flavored kefir also produced significant results, but they were less spectacular than the other three choices. Both the kefirs and yogurts reduced the severity of flatulence by 54 to 71 percent when compared with milk. Although the results for yogurt and kefir were similar, kefir is superior in terms of probiotics because it contains more species of beneficial bacteria than does yogurt. Therefore, even if you are not lactose intolerance, kefir is a great addition to your menu planning.

EAT PROBIOTICS DAILY!

Most probiotic foods have undergone at least partial fermentation, similar to the process that occurs in your gut among the bacteria. I recommend that you include at least a small portion of probiotic food at every meal. The list of probiotic foods is growing, as more and more food manufacturers are realizing the importance of beneficial bacteria in the diet. Therefore, expect to see many more functional foods on store shelves. Remember, the benefits derived from any probiotic food depend on the reliability of the production process, whether the product is shipped and stored properly, and whether you handle it properly once you get the food to your home. Always follow handling and storage instructions for any and all foods you buy.

PROBIOTIC FOODS
Acidophilus milk
Buttermilk
Sour cream (Some. Check label.)
Cottage cheese (Some. Check label.)
Miso dressings
Soft cheeses
Yogurt
Kefir
Sauerkraut (raw, cultured form)
Tempeh
Pickles and olives
Kimchee (pickled cabbage, radish, garlic, ginger,
and red pepper)

**Some less familiar probiotic foods (check local ethnic groceries
and on-line for these products):**
Laban rayab and laban zeer (Egyptian fermented milks)
Kishk (Egyptian fermented cereal and milk)
Gari (Nigerian fermented cassava)
Magou (South African fermented maize porridge)
Balao balao (Philippine fermented rice and shrimp)

Beneficial bacteria often found in probiotic foods:
Lactobacillus acidophilus, L. casei, L. johnsonii,
L. bulgaricus, L. rhamnosus, L. reuteri, Bifidobacterium lactis,
B. breve, B. animalis, B. infantis, B. longum,
Streptococcus thermophilus.

Making Yogurt

Yogurt making is an easy fermentation process that involves adding beneficial bacteria, primarily *Lactobacillus bulgaricus, L. acidophilus,* and *Streptococcus thermophilus,* to milk. The bacteria ferment the milk sugar (lactose) and transform it into lactic acid, which reduces the pH, causes the milk to curdle and turn tart, and also helps prevent the growth of bacteria that can cause food poisoning.

You can make yogurt at home using yogurt starter (available in health food stores, the natural foods section of some supermarkets, and on-line) or a live yogurt (a commercial brand that contains live cultures) as your starter culture. Since the fermentation process requires that you keep the developing yogurt at a constant temperature of around 110°F, you may want to purchase a yogurt maker. Here is a basic yogurt-making recipe.

- Bring one quart of milk (2% and whole milk work best) to a boil and then remove it from the heat and allow it to cool to 104–114°F. (Test with a candy thermometer.)
- Pour the milk into a sterile container and add one heaping tablespoon of live yogurt (or the appropriate amount of yogurt starter, as per package instructions).
- Stir the mixture well, cover, and incubate at 104–110°F for 6 to 10 hours, or until the yogurt is set. If you are using a yogurt maker, follow the instructions given with the machine.
- Refrigerate the yogurt once it has set.

PREBIOTICS AND OTHER PROBIOTIC HELPERS

Prebiotic Foods

Prebiotic foods are rich in soluble fiber, a nutrient that feeds and supports the development, growth, and function of beneficial bacteria in your gut. Prebiotic foods offer another benefit as well: They also help decrease the risk of cancer, diabetes, heart disease, stroke, hypertension, and obesity, plus they help keep your bowel function regular, which, as you've learned, is paramount to good health.

You may notice that there are many more prebiotic than probiotic foods, and that's the case for a very simple reason: Probiotic foods contain live organisms, and the shelf life of such foods is much shorter than that of prebiotics, which do not contain live bacteria. The lack of live bacteria in prebiotics also makes it easier for food manufacturers to add them to many food items, which expands the variety of prebiotic foods and in turn makes it easy to include prebiotic foods in your diet every day.

Eat Prebiotic Foods Daily!

See "Menu and Recipe Ideas" for help including these foods in your diet.

Artichokes
Bananas
Barley
Beans and legumes (black beans, chickpeas, kidney beans, lentils, navy beans, pinto beans, white beans)

Berries (esp. those with seeds—blackberries, blueberries, raspberries, strawberries)

Flax seed

Goats' milk

Greens (esp. dandelion, but also chard, collard, kale, mustard greens, spinach)

Miso

Oatmeal

Onions

Tomatoes

Whole grains

Bromelain Supplements

This pineapple derivative can have some potent, positive effects on your health, but it can also cause some minor negative responses in some people. If taking bromelain, consider these caveats:

- Bromelain may increase the risk of bleeding if it is taken along with drugs that increase bleeding, such as aspirin, warfarin, antiplatelet drugs (e.g., clopidogrel), and nonsteroidal anti-inflammatory drugs (NSAIDs). It may also increase bleeding risk if taken along with garlic, ginkgo biloba, or saw palmetto.

- Bromelain may increase the anti-inflammatory effects of NSAIDs.

- Bromelain may increase absorption of some antibiotics, including amoxicillin and tetracycline.

- When used along with ACE inhibitor drugs, bromelain may cause significant declines in blood pressure.

MSM Supplements

The natural organic sulfur compound, methylsulfonylmethane (MSM) is found in small amounts in many foods, especially fresh fruits and vegetables, but it is lost when food is processed. Even if you eat raw fruits and vegetables, you may still need to supplement with MSM, especially if you have certain conditions, such as asthma, allergies, arthritis, or digestive disorders.

As a supplement, MSM is odorless and virtually tasteless, with a slight bitterness. It is best taken as a powder (which can be mixed into your favorite beverages or soft foods) or capsule (which can be opened and the contents used as a powder). MSM rarely causes side effects, and if they do occur (e.g., nausea, headache, diarrhea), they typically disappear when you reduce the dose. Consult your physician before taking MSM if you are pregnant.

Sodium Chlorite

Sodium chlorite is available as a 5% solution that can cause a mild skin burn if it contacts the skin before it is diluted. One of the main functions of sodium chlorite is to help improve the efficiency of enzymes; another is to help resolve yeast infections. In these situations as well as others, a few drops of sodium chlorite solution is added to a glass of water and taken ninety minutes before or after your probiotic dose. Sources of sodium chlorite can be found in the appendix.

MENU AND RECIPE IDEAS

To give you an idea of the variety of probiotic and prebiotic foods that you can include in your diet, we have created a three-day menu plan that includes recipes (marked with an asterisk) for some of the items. We suggest you include both a probiotic supplement and probiotic food item at each meal. If that is not always possible, include one or the other at each meal.

✤ Three-Day Menu with Recipes

BREAKFAST:
Banana Smoothie*
Whole-grain bagel with all-natural peanut butter
Rooibos or decaf green tea

Banana Smoothie
Makes about 2 cups

8 oz. plain yogurt
½ cup acidophilus milk
1 medium banana, cut up

Place all ingredients in a blender and process until smooth.

LUNCH:
Tempting Tempeh Chili*
Sauerkraut Salad*
Herbal tea

Tempting Tempeh Chili
Makes 4 servings

2 tbs olive oil
8 oz. tempeh
2 cups cooked pinto, black, or kidney beans
1 large onion, diced
1 medium green pepper, seeded and diced

2½ cups tomato sauce

3 tbs chili powder (or to your taste)

1 tbs tamari

1 tbs dry mustard

1 tbs garlic powder

1 tsp cumin

Cut tempeh into small cubes and sauté in oil for about 10 minutes, until lightly browned. Add the rest of the ingredients and simmer for about 20 minutes. Serve over brown rice.

Sauerkraut Salad
Makes 4 servings

1½ lb. sauerkraut, rinsed and drained

3 green onions, sliced thin

3 tbs olive oil

1 cup pineapple, cut into small pieces (fresh preferred)

½ cup corn kernels

Wash, rinse, and drain the sauerkraut, and chop it if necessary. Place it in a large bowl and add the remaining ingredients. Toss well and then chill before serving.

DINNER:

Baked Chicken and Vegetables*

Mixed Greens Salad*

Kefir

Baked Chicken and Vegetables
Makes 4–5 servings

2 to 3 lbs chicken pieces
1 green bell pepper, cut into rings
2 medium onions, cut into 4 wedges each
4 small yams, halved
4 carrots, cut into 1-inch pieces
½ lb. fresh string beans, ends removed
2 cloves garlic, minced
1 Tbs. butter, melted
1 can (14–16 oz.) diced tomatoes
Salt and pepper to taste

Line a 9-×13-inch baking or roasting pan with foil. Arrange chicken, pepper rings, onions, garlic, yams, carrots, and string beans on the foil. Pour tomatoes over all and season with salt and pepper. Cover the pan with foil. Roast at 375°F for 1 hour or until vegetables are tender. Remove the foil, baste with juices, brush with melted butter, and continue roasting, uncovered, for about 30–40 minutes.

Mixed Greens Salad
Makes 4–6 servings

2 cups dandelion leaves, washed
2 cups fresh spinach, washed
2 cups romaine lettuce, washed
1 cucumber, peeled and sliced thin
3 tbs lemon juice

3 tbs olive oil
¼ tsp garlic powder
Salt and pepper to taste

Place all vegetables in a large bowl. Combine the remaining ingredients, mix well, and pour over the vegetables. Chill before serving if desired.

BREAKFAST:
Whole-grain cereal with yogurt topping
Fresh squeezed orange juice
Rooibos or decaf green tea

LUNCH:
Black and White Bean Soup*
Sourdough bread
Grain beverage

Black and White Bean Soup
Makes 4–6 servings

7 cups of vegetable broth or stock
1 can of white beans, rinsed and drained
1 can black beans, rinsed and drained
2 tbs olive oil
1 medium yellow onion, finely chopped
2 large carrots, finely chopped
1 celery stalk, finely chopped
2 cloves garlic, minced
1 tsp minced fresh or dried rosemary

Rinse the beans. In a large pot, heat the oil and sauté the onion, carrot, and celery until soft. Add the rosemary and garlic and sauté for 3 minutes. Add the beans and vegetable broth and bring to a boil. Reduce heat and simmer for 20 to 30 minutes. Place about ⅓ of the bean soup in a blender and process until smooth. (When blending hot soup, be sure to allow some of the steam and heat to escape every few seconds to avoid the lid blowing off the blender.) Return the blended soup to the pot and stir until well mixed. Serve.

DINNER:
Baked Flounder*
Barley Fiesta Salad*
Marinated veggies or kimchee
Herbal iced tea

Baked Flounder
Makes 4–6 servings

2 lb. flounder fillets, fresh or thawed (or comparable fish)
3 tomatoes, sliced
2 tbs flour
2 tbs butter
½ cup skim milk
⅓ cup dry white wine
Salt and pepper to taste
Garlic powder to taste
½ tsp dried basil

Sprinkle both sides of fish with salt, pepper, and garlic powder. Place fillets in a single layer in a greased baking dish. Arrange tomatoes on top of fillets. Sprinkle with salt, pepper, and garlic powder. Melt butter in sauce pan and blend in flour. Add milk gradually and cook until thick. Remove from heat and stir in wine and basil. Pour sauce over tomatoes. Bake in oven at 350°F for 25–30 minutes or until fish flakes easily.

Barley Fiesta Salad
Makes 8 servings

2 cups cooked barley
2 cups whole kernel corn
½ cup dried cranberries
¼ cup sliced green onions
1 unpeeled organic apple, chopped (about 1 cup)
1 carrot, shredded (about ⅓ cup)
2 tbs olive oil
2 tbs honey
1 tbs lemon juice

Combine all ingredients except the oil, honey, and lemon juice in a large bowl. Mix the oil, honey, and lemon juice in a shaker container and pour it over the barley mixture. Chill and serve.

BREAKFAST:
Free-range Egg Scramble w/ Veggies*
Whole-grain toast
Kefir

Free-Range Egg Scramble w/Veggies
Makes 2 servings

5 medium free-range eggs

2 tbs milk

2 slices onion, finely chopped

½ small green pepper, seeded and finely chopped

4 small fresh mushrooms, sliced

1 slice tomato, chopped

1 tbs butter

Salt and pepper to taste

Grated cheese (your choice)

In a medium bowl, beat the eggs, add milk, onions, peppers, and mushrooms. Melt butter in skillet over medium heat. Pour egg mixture into skillet. Scramble lightly. Remove from heat, divide into servings, and top with chopped tomatoes and cheese. Cover and allow cheese to melt.

LUNCH:

Creamy Potato Soup*

Fresh berries w/sour cream (with active cultures)

Herbal tea

Creamy Potato Soup

1 tbs olive oil

2 cups plain kefir

2 cups diced sweet onion

2 cups peeled, diced yams

1 cup peeled diced white potatoes

4 cups vegetable broth

2 cloves garlic

Salt and pepper to taste

Dash of cumin

Heat the oil in a large soup pot. Add the onions and garlic and sauté for 3–4 minutes. Add the yams, potatoes, and broth. Bring to a boil, reduce heat, and simmer for 25–30 minutes. Puree the soup and season with salt, pepper, and cumin. Whisk in the kefir and serve.

DINNER:

Whole-grain Pasta with Mushroom*

Marinated artichoke hearts and olives

Tomato juice w/lemon slice

Whole-Grain Pasta w/Mushroom Sauce

Makes 4 servings

8 oz. whole-wheat pasta

4 oz. mushrooms (shiitake, brown—your choice)

1 tbs butter

2 cloves garlic, minced

¼ cup cottage cheese (with live cultures)

¼ cup low-fat milk

¼ cup grated parmesan

Salt and pepper to taste

Prepare pasta according to package directions. In the meantime, clean the mushrooms and cut into ¼-inch slices. Melt the butter in a large skillet and add the mushrooms and garlic. Cover the skillet and allow the mushrooms to simmer until they are tender (about 15 minutes). Combine the cottage cheese, milk, and parmesan in a blender and blend until smooth. Drain the pasta and add it to the mushroom mixture. Add the cottage cheese mixtures and return the skillet to low heat. Season with salt and pepper and toss the pasta until it is evenly coated.

Notes

List of Abbreviations

Acta Univ Carol [Med] (Praha) — ACTA Universitatis Carolinae. Medica (Praha)

Agric Biol Chem — Agricultural and Biological Chemistry

Aliment Pharmacol Ther — Alimentary Pharmacology and Therapeutics

Altern Med Rev — Alternative Medicine Review

Amer Diet Assoc — American Dietetic Association

Am J Clin Nutr — American Journal of Clinical Nutrition

Am J Epidemiology — American Journal of Epidemiology

Am J Gastroenterol — American Journal of Gastroenterology

Ann Epidemiol — Annals of Epidemiology

Ann Surg — Annals of Surgery

Appl Environ Microbiol — Applied and Environmental Microbiology

Arch Dis Child — Archives of Disease in Childhood

Arch Fam Med — Archives of Family Medicine

Baillieres Clin Gastroenterol — Baillieres Clinical Gastroenterology

Bifidobacteria & Microflora — Bifidobacteria & Microflora

Biomed Pharmacother — Biomedicine and Pharmacotherapy

B J Dermatol — British Journal of Dermatology

BMJ	*British Medical Journal*
Br J Gen Pract	*British Journal of General Practice*
Br J Nutr	*British Journal of Nutrition*
Bratisl Lek Listy	*Bratislavske Lekarske Listy*
Cancer Chemother Pharmacol	*Cancer Chemotherapy and Pharmacology*
Cas Lek Cesk	*Casopis Lekaru Ceskych*
Clin Exp Allergy	*Clinical and Experimental Allergy*
Clin Inf Dis	*Clinical Infectious Diseases*
Clin Nutr Insights	*Clinical Nutrition Insights*
Clin Ped	*Clinical Pediatrics*
CRC Crit Rev Food Sci Nutr	*CRC Critical Reviews in Food Science and Nutrition*
Curr Gastroenterol Rep	*Current Gastroenterology Reports*
Curr Sci	*Current Science*
Dig Dis Sci	*Digestive Diseases and Sciences*
Environ Health Perspect	*Environmental Health Perspectives*
Eur J Clin Nutr	*European Journal of Clinical Nutrition*
Eur J Oral Sci	*European Journal of Oral Sciences*
Eur Urol	*European Urology*
FEBS Lett	*FEBS Letters*
FEMS Immunol Med Microbiol	*FEMS Immunology and Medical Microbiology*
FEMS Microbiol Lett	*FEMS Microbiology Letters*
Gastroenterol Clin North Am	*Gastroenterology Clinics of North America*
Gastroenterol Hepatol	*Gastroenterologia y Hepatologia*
Infect Immun	*Infection and Immunity*
Int J Antimicro Ag	*International Journal of Antimicrobial Agents*
Int J Epidemiology	*International Journal of Epidemiology*
J Allergy Clin Immunol	*Journal of Allergy and Clinical Immunology*
J Am Den Assoc	*Journal of the American Dental Association*
J Am Diet Assoc	*Journal of the American Dietetic Association*
J Antimicrob Chemother	*Journal of Antimicrobial Chemotherapy*

J Appl Bacteriol	*Journal of Applied Bacteriology*
J Appl Microbiol	*Journal of Applied Microbiology*
J Bone Miner Res	*Journal of Bone and Mineral Research*
J Clin Gastroenterol	*Journal of Clinical Gastroenterology*
J Clin Immun	*Journal of Clinical Immunology*
J Dairy Sci	*Journal of Dairy Science*
J Dairy Res	*Journal of Dairy Research*
J Dent Res	*Journal of Dental Research*
J Nutr	*Journal of Nutrition*
J Pediatr	*Journal of Pediatrics*
J Pediatr Gastroenterol Nutr	*Journal of Pediatrics Gastroenterology and Nutrition*
J Periodontol	*Journal of Periodontology*
J Urol	*Journal of Urology*
Langenbecks Arch Chir	*Langenbecks Archiv fur Chirurgie*
Mater Med Pol	*Materia Medica Polona*
Med Dosw Mikrobiol	*Medycyna Doswiadczalna I Mikrobiologia*
Microb Ecol	*Microbial Ecology*
Microb Ecology Health Dis	*Microbial Ecology in Health and Disease*
MMW Fortschr Med	*Fortschritte der Medizin*
Mol Biother	*Molecular Biotherapy*
NEJM	*New England Journal of Medicine*
Nutr Res	*Nutrition Reviews*
Nutr Cancer	*Nutrition and Cancer*
Occup Environ Med	*Occupational and Environmental Medicine*
Pediatr Infect Dis J	*Pediatric Infectious Disease Journal*
Periodontol	*Periodontology 200*
PDR	*Physicians' Desk Reference*
Postgrad Med J	*Postgraduate Medical Journal*
Prescrire Int	*Prescrire International*
Proc Soc Exp Biol Med	*Proceedings of the Society for Experimental Biology and Medicine*
Scand J Nutr	*Scandinavian Journal of Nutrition*
Sci	*Science*
Stomotologiia	*Stomotologiia*
Swed Dent J	*Swedish Dental Journal*

Urol Int	*Urologia Internationalis*
World J Urol	*World Journal of Urology*
World J Gastroenterol	*World Journal of Gastroenterology*
Z Gastroenterol	*Zeitschrift fur Gastroenterologie*

1. Why Everyone Needs Probiotics

Bengmark S. Colonic food: pre- and probiotics. *Am J Gastroenterol* 2000; 95:S5–S7.

Bjorksten B. Evidence of probiotics in prevention of allergy and asthma. *Curr Drug Targets Inflamm Allergy* 2005 Oct; 4(5):599–604.

Drisko, J. A. et al. Probiotics in health maintenance and disease prevention. *Altern Med Rev* 2003 May; 8(2):143–55.

Macfarlane, G.T. and H.J. Cummings. Probiotics and prebiotics: Can regulating the activities of intestinal bacteria benefit health? *BJM* 1999; 318:999–1003.

Mercola, J. and R. Droege. 100 Trillion Bacteria in Your Gut: Learn How to Keep the Good Kind There.

Physicians Drug Reference Web site: www.pdrhealth.com/drug-info/ nmdrugprofiles/nutsupdrugs/pro_0034.shtml.

Vanderhoof, J. A. "Probiotics and inflammatory disorders in infants and children." *J Ped Gastroenterol Nutr* 2000; 30:S34–S38.

2. Probiotics: An Inside Look at How They Work

Bengmark, S. Colonic food: pre- and probiotics. *Am J Gastroenterol* 2000; 95:S5–S7.

Bogdanov, I. G. et al. Antitumor glycopeptides from lactobacillus bulgaricus cell wall. 1975; *FEBS Lett* 57:259.

Clemmesen, J. Antitumor effect of lactobacilli substances: L. bulgaricus effect. *Mol Biother* 1989 1(5): 279–82.

Deguchi, Y. et al. Comparative studies on synthesis of water-soluble vitamins among human species of bifidobacteria. *Agric Biol Chem* 1985; 49:13–19.

Gibson, G. R. et al. Gastrointestinal microbial disease and probiotics. In: Fuller, R., ed. *Probiotics: Therapeutic and Other Beneficial Effects.* London: Chapman and Hall, 1997:10–39.

Grahn, E. et al. Interference of a Lactococcus lactis strain on the human gut flora and its capacity to pass the stomach and intestine. *Scand J Nutr* 1994; 38: 2–4.

Guslandi, M. et al. Saccharomyces boulardii in maintenance treatment of Crohn's disease. *Dig Dis Sci* 2000; 45:1462–64.

Hlivak, P. et al. One-year application of probiotic strain Enterococcus faecium M-74 decreases serum cholesterol levels. *Bratisl Lek Listy* 2005; 106(2): 67–72.

Kimoto, H. et al. Cholesterol removal from media by Lactococci. *J Dairy Sci* 2002; 85:3182–88.

Klijn, N. et al. Genetic marking of Lactococcus lactis shows its survival in the human gastrointestinal tract. *Appl Environ Microbiol* 1995; 61:2771–74.

Metchnikoff, E. *The Prolongation of Life: Optimistic Studies.* New York: G.P. Putnam's Sons 1908.

Pompei, A. et al. Folate production by Bifidobacteria as a potential probiotic property. *Appl Environ Microbiol* Jan. 2007; 73(1): 179–85.

http://www.pdrhealth.com/drug_info/nmdrugprofiles/nutsupdrugs/pro_0034.shtml.

3. Prebiotics and Other Probiotic Helpers

Agheli, N. et al. Plasma lipids and fatty acid synthase activity are regulated by short-chain fructooligosaccharides in sucrose-fed, insulin-resistant rats. *J Nutr* 1998; 128:1283–8.

Bovee-Oudenhover, I. M. et al. Increasing the intestinal resistance of rats to the invasive pathogen Salmonella enteritidis: additive effects of dietary lactulose and calcium. *Gut* 1997 Apr; 40(4):497–504.

Commane, D. M. et al. Effects of fermentation products of pro- and prebiotics on trans-epithelial electrical resistance in an in vitro model of the colon. *Nutr Cancer* 2005; 51(1):102–9.

Crittenden, R. G. *Prebiotics—A Critical Review.* Horizon Scientific Press. ISBN 1-898486-15-8 1999; 10:141–156.

Delzenne, N. and N. Kok, et al. Dietary fructooligosaccharides modify lipid metabolism in the rat. *Am J Clin Nutr* 1993; 57:Suppl 820.

Djouzi, Z. and C. Andrieux. Compared effects of three oligosaccharides on metabolism of intestinal microflora in rats inoculated with a human faecal flora. *Br J Nutr* 1997; 78:313–24.

Fiordaliso, M. et al. Dietary oligofructose lowers triglycerides, phospholipids, and cholesterol in serum and very low-density lipoproteins in rats. *Lipids* 1995; 30:163–67.

Huchzermeyer, H. and C. Schumann. Lactulose—a multifaceted substance. *Z Gastroenterol* 1997 Oct; 35(10): 945–55.

International Food Information Council: www.ific.org/foodinsight/2003/ma/friendlybugsfi203.cfm.

Jackson, K. G. et al. The effect of the daily intake of inulin on fasting lipid, insulin, and glucose concentrations in middle-aged men and women. *Br J Nutr* 1999 Jul; 82(1):23–30.

LeLeu, R. K. et al. A synbiotic combination of resistant starch and Bifidobacterium lactis facilitates apoptotic deletion of carcinogen-damaged cells in rat colon. *J Nutr* 2005 May; 135(5):996–1001.

Letexier, D. et al. Addition of inulin to a moderately high-carbohydrate diet reduces hepatic lipogenesis and plasma triacylglycerol concentrations in humans. *Am J Clin Nutr* 2003 Mar; 77(3): 559–64.

Macfarlane, G. T. and J. H. Cummings. Probiotics and prebiotics: Can regulating the activities of intestinal bacteria benefit health? *BMJ* April 10, 1999; 318:999–1003.

Moshfegh, A. J. et al. Presence of inulin and oligofructose in the diet of Americans. *J Nutr* 1999 129:75.

Nouza, K. Outlooks of systemic enzyme therapy in rheumatoid arthritis and other immunopathological diseases. *Acta Univ Carol [Med]* (Praha). 1994; 40(1–4):101–4.

Pool-Zobel, B. L. Inulin-type fructans and reduction in colon cancer risk: Review of experimental and human data. *Br J Nutr* 2005 Apr; 93 Suppl 1:S73–90.

Roberfroid, M. B. Prebiotics and probiotics: Are they functional foods? *Am J Clin Nutr* 2000; 71 (6 Suppl):1682S–1690S.

Rycroft, C. E. et al. A comparative in vitro evaluation of the fermentation properties of prebiotic oligosaccharides. *J Appl Microbiol* 2001 91:878–87.

Stauder, G. Pharmacological effects of oral enzyme combinations. *Cas Lek Cesk* 1995 Oct 4; 134(19):620–24.

Stauder, G. et al. The use of hydrolytic enzymes as adjuvant therapy in AIDS/ARC/LAS patients. *Biomed Pharmacother* 1988; 42(1): 31–34.

Tahiri, M. et al. Five-week intake of short-chain fructooligosaccharides increases intestinal absorption and status of magnesium in postmenopausal women. *J Bone Miner Res* 2001 16:2152–60.

Van den Heuvel, E. G. et al. Lactulose stimulates calcium absorption in postmenopausal women. *J Bone Miner Res* 1999 Jul; 14(7): 1211–16.

Van Loo, J. et al. On the presence of inulin and oligofructose as natural ingredients in the Western diet. *CRC Crit Rev Food Sci Nutr* 1995; 35:525–52.

Verghese, M. et al. Dietary inulin suppresses azoxymethane-induced aberrant crypt foci and colon tumors at the promotion stage in young Fisher 344 rats. *J Nutr* 2002 Sep; 132(9): 2809–13.

Wang, X. and G. R. Gibson. Effects of the in vitro fermentation of oligofructose and inulin by bacteria growing in the human large intestine. *J Appl Bacteriol* 1993 75:373–80.

Williams, C. M. and K. F. Jackson. Inulin and oligofructose: effects on lipid metabolism from human studies. *Br J Nutr* 2002 May; 87 Suppl 2:S261–64.

Wollowski, I. et al. Protective role of probiotics and prebiotics in colon cancer. *Am J Clin Nutr* 2001 Feb; 73(2 Suppl):451S–455S.

Wong, J. M. et al. Colonic health: fermentation and short-chain fatty acids. *J Clin Gastroenterol* 2006 Mar; 40(3):235–43.

4. The Core Program: Building a Better You

Cantor, K. P. et al. Drinking water source and chlorination by-products. I. Risk of bladder cancer. *Epidemiology* 1998 Jan; 9(1):21–28.

Fackelmann, K. A. Hints of a chlorine cancer connection. *Science News* July 11, 1992; 142:23.

Flaten, T. P. Chlorination of drinking water and cancer incidence in Norway. *Intl J Epidemiology* 1992; 21(1): 6–15.

Koivusalo, M. et al. Drinking water mutagenicity and urinary tract cancers: A population-based case-control study in Finland. *Am J Epidemiol* 1998 Oct 1;148(7):704–12.

Morris, R. D. Chlorination, chlorination by-products, and cancer. *Am J Public Health* July 1992; 82(7): 955–63.

———. Drinking water and cancer. *Environ Health Perspect.* 1995 Nov; 103 Suppl 8:225–31.

National Sleep Foundation 2001, 2002, & 2004. Sleep in America poll results: see www.sleepfoundation.org

Nickmilder, M. and A. Bernard. Ecological association between childhood asthma and availability of indoor chlorinated swimming pools in Europe. *Occup Environ Med* 2007 Jan; 64(1):37–46.

Olivares, M. et al. Dietary deprivation of fermented foods causes a fall in innate immune response. Lactic acid bacteria can counteract the immunological effect of this deprivation. *J Dairy Res* 2006 Nov; 73(4):492–8. Epub 2006 Sep 21.

Rothery, S. P. et al. Hazards of chlorine to asthmatic patients. *Br J Gen Pract* Jan. 1991:39.

Shahani, K. *Cultivate Health From Within*, p. 25; original source, Wiley, T.S. and Bent Formby, *Lights Out!* New York: Pocket Books, 2000, pp. 48–51, 53.

Zareie, M. et al. Probiotics prevent bacterial translocation and improve intestinal barrier function in rats following chronic psychological stress. *Gut* 2006 Nov; 55(11):1553–60. Epub 2006 Apr 25.

5. Gastrointestinal Problems

Bibiloni, R. et al. VSL#3 probiotic mixture induces remission in patients with active ulcerative colitis. *Am J Gastroenterol* 2005; 100: 1539–46.

Bohn, S. Kruis. Probiotics in chronic inflammatory bowel disease. *MMW Fortschr Med* 2006 Aug 31; 148 (35–36): 30–34.

Buchman, A. L., ed. Book review, *Clinical Nutrition in Gastrointestinal Diseases*, in *NEJM* 2007 Feb. 14; 356(7): 758–59.

Campieri, M. et al. Combination of antibiotic and probiotic treatment is efficacious in prophylaxis of postoperative recurrence of Crohn's disease: A randomized controlled study vs. mesalazine. *Gastroenterology* 2000; 118:A781.

Chapman, T. M. et al. Spotlight on VSL#3 probiotic mixture in chronic inflammatory bowel diseases. *BioDrugs* 2007; 21(1):61–63.

Gaynes, B. N. and D. A. Drossman. The role of psychosocial factors in irritable bowel syndrome. *Baillieres Clin Gastroenterol* 1999; 13(3):437–52.

Gionchetti, P. et al. Antibiotics and probiotics in treatment of inflammatory bowel disease. *World J Gastroenterol* 2006 June 7; 12(21): 3306–13.

Guslandi, M. et al. Saccharomyces boulardii in maintenance treatment of Crohn's disease. *Dig Dis Sci* 2000; 45:1462–64.

Histamine-2 receptor antagonists and proton pump inhibitors reduce B12 absorption. *Arch Fam Med* 1999; 8:271.

Huebner, E. S. and C. M. Surawicz. Treatment of recurrent Clostridium difficile diarrhea. *Gastroentero Hepatology* 2006; 2, 203–8.

McFarland, L. V. Meta-analysis of probiotics for the prevention of antibiotic-associated diarrhea and the treatment of Clostridium difficile disease. *Am J Gastroenterol* 2006; 101, 812–22.

National Institutes of Health, "Irritable bowel syndrome," publication #06-693, 2006.

Rinne, M. et al. Effect of probiotics and breastfeeding on the bifidobacterium and lactobacillus/enterococcus microbiota and humoral immune responses. *J Pediatr* 2005 Aug; 147(2):186–91.

Thompson, W. G. et al. Functional bowel disorders and functional abdominal pain. *Gut* 1999; 45:43–47.

Venturi, A. et al. Impact on the composition of the faecal flora by a new probiotic preparation: preliminary data on maintenance treatment of patients with ulcerative colitis. *Aliment Pharmacol Ther* 1999; 13: 1103–8.

Wenus, C. et al. Prevention of antibiotic-associated diarrhoea by a fermented probiotic milk drink. *Eur J Clin Nutr* 2007 Mar 14.

Yang, Y.-X. et al. Long-term proton pump inhibitor therapy and risk of hip fracture. *JAMA* 2006; 296:2947–53.

6. Allergies and Athsma

American Academy of Allergy, Asthma and Immunology (AAAAI). *The Allergy Report: Science-Based Findings on the Diagnosis & Treatment of Allergic Disorders,* 1996–2001.

Boguniewicz, M. and D. Leung. *In Allergy, Principles and Practice,* 5th Ed., E. Middleton et al, ed. Mosby, St. Louis, p. 1123. 1998.

Folster-Holst, R. et al. Prospective, randomized, controlled trial on Lactobacillus rhamnosus in infants with moderate to severe atopic dermatitis. *Br J Dermatol* 2006; 155:1256–61.

Hauer, A. Probiotics in allergic diseases of childhood. *MMW Fortschr Med* 2006 Aug 31; 148(35–36): 34–36.

Horan, R. F. et al. Allergic disorders and mastocytosis. *JAMA* 1992; 268:2858–68.

Isolauri, E. et al. Probiotics in the management of atopic eczema. *Clin Exp Allergy.* 2000; 30:1604–10.

Kirjavainen, P. V. et al. Probiotic bacteria in the management of atopic disease: underscoring the importance of viability. *J Pediatr Gastroenterol Nutr* 2003; 36:223–27.

Larsen, F. and J. Hanikin. Epidemiology of atopic dermatitis. *Immunol Allergy Clin NA* 2002; 22:1–25.

Majamaa, H. and E. Isolauri. Probiotics: a novel approach in the management of food allergy. *J Allergy Clin Immunol* 1997; 99:179–85.

Moro, G. et al. A mixture of prebiotic oligosaccharides reduces the incidence of atopic dermatitis during the first six months of age. *Arch Dis Child* 2006 Oct; 91(10): 814–19.

Natahn, R. A. et al. Prevalence of allergic rhinitis in the United States. *J Aller Clin Immunol* 1997; 99:S808–14.

Rosenfeldt, V. et al. Effect of probiotic Lactobacillus strains in children with atopic dermatitis. *J Allergy Clin Immunol* 2003; 111:389–95.

Rudikoff, D. and M. Lebwohl. Atopic dermatitis. 1998; *Lancet* 351(9117): 1715–21.

Sampson, H. A. Peanut allergy. *NEJM* 2002; 346:1294–99.

Sicherer, S. H. et al. Prevalence of peanut and tree nut allergy in the United States determined by means of a random digit dial telephone survey: A 5-year follow-up study. *J Allergy Clin Immunol* 2003; 112(6):1203–7.

———. Prevalence of seafood allergy in the United States determined by a random telephone survey. *J Allergy Clin Immunol* 2004; 114:159–65.

Taylor, A. L. et al. Probiotic supplementation for the first 6 months of life fails to reduce the risk of atopic dermatitis and increases the risk of allergen sensitization in high-risk children: a randomized controlled trial. *J Allergy Clin Immunol* 2007; 119:184–91.

Viljanen, M. et al. Probiotics in the treatment of atopic eczema/ dermatitis syndrome in infants: a double-blind placebo-controlled trial. *Allergy* 2005; 60:494–500.

Weston, S. et al. Effects of probiotics on atopic dermatitis: a randomised controlled trial. *Arch Dis Child.* 2005 Apr 29.

7. Reproductive and Urinary Tract Infections

Ambulatory Care Visits to Physician Offices, Hospital Outpatient Departments, and Emergency Departments: United States, 1999–2000. Vital and Health Statistics. Series 13, No. 157. Hyattsville, MD: National Center for Health Statistics, CDC, U.S. Dept. of Health and Human Services; September 2004.

Anukam, K. C. et al. Clinical study comparing probiotic Lactobacillus GR-1 and RC-14 with metronidazole vaginal gel to treat symptomatic bacterial vaginosis. *Microbes Infect.* 2006 Oct; 8(12–13):2772–76.

Cadieux, R. et al. Lactobacillus strains and vaginal ecology. *JAMA* 2002; 287:1940–1941.

Falagas, M. E. et al. Probiotics for prevention of recurrent vulvovaginal candidiasis: a review. *J Antimicrob Chemother* 2006 Aug; 58(2): 266–72.

———. Probiotics for prevention of recurrent urinary tract infections in women: A review of the evidence from microbiological and clinical studies. *Drugs* 2006; 66(9): 1253–61.

Foxman, B. et al. Urinary tract infection: self-reported incidence and associated costs. *Ann Epidemiol* 2000; 10:509–15.

Kontiokari, T. et al. Dietary factors protecting women from urinary tract infections. *Am J Clin Nutr* 2003 Mar; 77(3): 600–4.

Kwok, L. et al. Adherence of Lactobacillus crispatus to vaginal epithelial cells from women with or without a history of recurrent urinary tract infection. *J Urol* 2006 Nov; 176(5): 2050–54.

Lactobacillus sporogenes monograph. *Altern Med Rev* 2002; 7:340–42.

Lemar, K. M. et al. Garlic (Allium sativum) as an anti-Candida agent: a comparison of the efficacy of fresh garlic and freeze-dried extracts. *J Appl Microbiol* 2002; 93:398–405.

Marrazzo, J. M. et al. Women's satisfaction with an intravaginal Lactobacillus capsule for the treatment of bacterial vaginosis. *J Womens Health* 2006 Nov; 15(9): 1053–60.

Pascual, L. M. et al. Lactobacillus species isolated from the vagina: identification, hydrogen peroxide production and nonoxynol-9 resistance. *Contraception* 2006 Jan; 73(1): 78–81.

Reid, G. and A. W. Bruce. Probiotics to prevent urinary tract infections: the rationale and evidence. *World J Urol* 2006 Feb; 24(1): 28–32.

Reid, G. et al. Oral probiotics can resolve urogenital infections. *FEMS Immunol Med Microbiol* 2001 Feb; 30(1): 49–52.

Strus, M. et al. Inhibitory activity of vaginal Lactobacillus bacteria on yeast-causing vulvovaginal candidiasis. *Med Dosw Mikrobiol* 2005; 57(1): 7–17.

Uehara, S. et al. A pilot study evaluating the safety and effectiveness of Lactobacillus vaginal suppositories in patients with recurrent urinary tract infection. *Int J Antimicrob Ag.* 2006 Aug; 28 Suppl 1:S30.

Vanderhoof, J. A. and R. J. Young. Use of probiotics in childhood gastrointestinal disorders. *J Pediatr Gastroenterol Nutr* 1998; 27:323–32.

8. The Immune System

Aso, Y. and H. Akazan. Prophylactic effect of a Lactobacillus casei preparation on the recurrence of superficial bladder cancer. BLP Study Group. *Urol Int* 1992; 49:125–29.

Aso, Y. et al. Preventive effect of a Lactobacillus casei preparation on the recurrence of superficial bladder cancer in a double-blind trial. The BLP Study Group. *Eur Urol* 1995; 27;104–9.

Capurso, G. et al. Probiotics and the incidence of colorectal cancer: when evidence is not evident. *Dig Liver Dis* 2006 Dec; 38 Suppl 2:S277–82.

deVrese, M. et al. Probiotic bacteria reduced duration and severity but not the incidence of common cold episodes in a double-blind, randomized, controlled trial. *Vaccine.* 2006 Nov 10; 24(44–46):6670–74. Epub 2006 Jun 6.

Femia, A. P. et al. Antitumorigenic activity of the prebiotic inulin enriched with oligofructose in combination with the probiotics Lactobacillus rhamnosus and Bifidobacterium lactis on azoxymethane-induced colon carcinogenesis in rats. *Carcinogenesis* 2002; 23:1953–60.

Gill, H. S. et al. Enhancement of immunity in the elderly by dietary supplementation with the probiotic Bifidobacterium lactis HN019. *Am J Clin Nutr* 74, 6:833–39, 2001.

———. Dietary probiotic supplementation enhances natural killer cell activity in the elderly: an investigation of age-related immunological changes. *J Clin Immunol* 21, 4:264–71, 2001.

Gorbach, S. L. Probiotics and gastrointestinal health. *Am J Gastroenterol* 2000; 95:S2–S4.

Gorbach, S. L. and B. R. Goldin. Nutrition and the gastrointestinal microflora. *Nutr Res* 1992; 50:378–81.

Hooper, L. V. and J. I. Gordon. Commensal host-bacterial relationships in the gut. *Science* 2001:292:1115–18.

Kanazawa, H. et al. Synbiotics reduce postoperative infections complications: a randomized controlled trial in biliary cancer patients undergoing hepatectomy. *Langenbecks Arch Chir* 2005 Apr. 390(2): 104–13.

Keswani, R. N. and R. D. Cohen. Postoperative management of ulcerative colitis and Crohn's disease. *Curr Gastroenterol Rep.* 2005 Dec; 7(6):492–99.

Okumura, A. et al. Oseltamivir and delirious behavior in children with influenza. *Pediatr Infect Dis J* 2006 Jun; 25(6):572.

Oseltamivir: cutaneous and neurological adverse effects in children. *Prescrire Int* 2006 Oct; 15(85):182–83.

Percival, M. Choosing a probiotic supplement. *Clin Nutr Insights* 1997;6:1–4.

Sakalova, A. et al. Retrolective cohort study of an additive therapy with an oral enzyme preparation in patients with multiple myeloma. *Cancer Chemother Pharmacol* 2001; 47:S38–44.

Sarem-Damerdji, L. et al. In vitro colonization ability of human colon mucosa by exogenous Lactobacillus strains. *FEMS Microbiol Lett* 1995; 131:133–37.

Sugawara, G. et al. Perioperative symbiotic treatment to prevent postoperative infection complications in biliary cancer surgery: a randomized controlled trial. *Ann Surg* 2006 Nov; 244(5): 706–14.

Vanderhoof, J. A. Probiotics: future directions. *Am J Clin Nutr* 2001; 73:1152S–1155S.

Vanderhoof, J. A. and R. J. Young. Use of probiotics in childhood gastrointestinal disorders. *J Pediatr Gastroenterol Nutr* 1998;27:323–32.

Walker, W. A. Role of nutrients and bacterial colonization in the development of intestinal host defense. *J Pediatr Gastroenterol Nutr* 2000;30:S2–S7.

9. Weight Management

Kimoto, H. et al. Cholesterol removal from media by Lactococci. *J Dairy Sci* 2002; 85:3182–88.

Lactobacillus sporogenes monograph. *Altern Med Rev* 2002; 7:340–42. See article at www.findarticles.com/p/articles/mi_m0FDN/is_2_8/ai_103377069/pg_1

Sanders, M. E. and T. R. Klaenhammer. Invited review: the scientific basis of Lactobacillus acidophilus NCFM functionality as a probiotic. *J Dairy Sci* 2001;84:319–31.

Survarna, V. C. and V. U. Boby. Probiotics in human health: A current assessment. *Current Science* 2005; 88(11): 1744–48.

University of Michigan Health Systems press release: "Probiotic microbes could be a key to good health." March 6, 2006; at www.med.umich.edu/opm/newspage/2006/hmprobiotics.htm

10. The Aging Challenge

Dreiling, D. A. et al. Human exocrine pancreatic secretion changes associated with age. *Mater Med Pol* 2000; 17–19.

Hamilton-Miller, J. M. T. Probiotics and prebiotics in the elderly. *Postgrad Med J* 2004; 80:447–51.

Hayakawa, K. et al. Effects of soybean oligosaccharides on human faecal microflora. *Microb Ecology Health Dis* 1990; 3:293–303.

Hidaka, H., T. Eida, et al. Effects of fructooligosaccharides on intestinal flora and human health. *Bifidobacteria and Microflora* 1986; 5:37–50.

Majumdar, A. P. N. et al. Effect of aging on the gastrointestinal tract and the pancreas. *Proc Soc Exp Biol Med* 1997; 215.

Saunier, K. and J. Dore. Gastrointestinal tract and the elderly: functional foods, gut microflora and healthy aging. *Dig Liver Dis* 2002 Sep; 34 Suppl 2:S19–24.

Tuohy, K. M. et al. Using probiotics and prebiotics to improve gut health. *Drug Discov Today* 2003 Aug 1; 8(15): 692–700.

11. Better Oral Health

Barnett, M. L. The rationale for the daily use of an antimicrobial mouthrise. *J Am Dent Assoc* 2006; 137(3):16S–21S.

Cagler, E. et al. Bacteriotherapy and probiotics' role in oral health. *Oral Diseases* 2005 May; 11(3): 131–37.

Grudianov, A. I. et al. Use of probiotics Bifidumbacterin and Acilact in tablets in therapy of periodontal inflammations. *Stomatologiia (Mosk)* 2002; 81(1): 39–43.

Hart, G. T. et al. Quantitative gene expression profiling implicates genes for susceptibility and resistance to alveolar bone loss. *Infect Immun* 2004; 72(8): 4471–79.

Hatakka, K. et al. Probiotics reduce the prevalence of oral candida in the elderly: a randomized controlled trial. *J Dent Res* 2007 Feb; 86(2): 125–30.

Kinane, D. F. et al. The genetic basis of periodontitis. *Periodontol 2000* 2005; 39:91–117.

Krasse, P. et al. Decreased gum bleeding and decreased gingivitis by the probiotic Lactobacillus reuteri. *Swed Dent J* 2006; 30(2): 55–60.

Meurman, J. H. Probiotics: do they have a role in oral medicine and dentistry? *Eur J Oral Sci* 2005 Jun; 113(3): 188–96.

Mongardini, C. et al. One-stage full- versus partial-mouth disinfection in the treatment of chronic adult or generalized early-onset periodontitis, I: long-term clinical observations. *J Periodontol* 1999; 70(6):632–45.

Quirynen, M. et al. Full- vs. partial-mouth disinfection in the treatment of periodontal infections: short-term clinical and microbiological observations. *J Dent Res* 1995; 74(8):1459–67.

Wilson, W. et al. Prevention of infective endocarditis. Guidelines from the American Heart Association, *Circ* 2007 Apr 19 (Epub ahead of print).

12. How to Choose and Use Probiotics and Their Helpers

Heller, K. J. Probiotic bacteria in fermented foods: product characteristics and starter organisms. *Am J Clin Nutr* 2001; 73(2): 374S–79S.

Hertzler, S. M. and S. R. Clancy. Kefir improves lactose digestion and tolerance in adults with lactose maldigestion. *J Am Diet Assoc* 2003 May; 103(5): 582–87.

Glossary

Acidophilus: One of many species of good bacteria belonging to the genus *Lactobacillus*. Acidophilus inhabits the gastrointestinal tract and produces natural antibiotics, including acidolphin, lactophilin, and bacteriocidin, that help destroy bad bacteria.

Aerobic: Bacteria that need oxygen to grow, reproduce, and function.

Amylase: An enzyme that helps transform starches or complex carbohydrates into smaller units of sugar.

Anaerobic: Bacteria that can grow, reproduce, and function in the absence of oxygen.

Antigen: A substance that causes the body to produce an antibody and that may or may not result in an allergic reaction.

Bifidobacterium: A family of friendly bacteria that inhabit the large intestine of adults and the digestive tract and feces of infants.

Candida albicans: A yeast that is normally found in the human body, especially on the skin and mucus membranes. An overgrowth of *Candida* is called candidiasis.

Coenzyme: A small, nonprotein substance that enhances the actions of an enzyme.

Dysbiosis: A condition in which the bacterial population of the gut is out of balance.

Enzyme: Any protein that has the ability to regulate chemical reactions in the body. Enzymes are necessary for life.

Fermentation: A process by which certain bacteria, yeasts, and molds cause a chemical change in a substance (e.g., milk) in the absence of oxygen and produces energy.

Flora: A collection of bacteria, yeasts, and other microorganisms that occur on or within the body; for example, the intestinal bacterial flora.

Fructooligosaccharide (FOS): A type of carbohydrate, and more specifically, complex groups of sugar molecules that serve as food for beneficial bacteria in the gut.

Inulin: A type of carbohydrate (specifically, a fiber) found in plants, that serves as "food" (i.e., a prebiotic) for the beneficial bacteria in the gut.

Irritable bowel syndrome: A gastrointestinal disorder characterized by a highly sensitive colon, bloating, alternative bouts of diarrhea and constipation, and abdominal pain. It is considered a functional disorder because there are no signs of disease when the colon is examined.

Lactic acid: A substance that occurs in three forms: L, D, and DL. The L form is produced in muscle during exercise; D is formed by fermentation of dextrose by microorganisms; and DL is found in the stomach and in certain fermented foods.

Lactose: A sugar in milk that yields glucose and galactose when it is broken down.

Lactose intolerance: An inability to properly metabolize lactose.

Lipase: An enzyme that breaks down fats into fatty acids and glycerol.

Peptidase: An enzyme that initiates the breakdown of peptides into amino acids.

pH: The representation of hydrogen ion concentration of a substance. It is measured on a scale of 1 to 14, with 7 being neutral. Numbers lower than 7 indicate that a substance has more acidity; numbers greater than 7 indicate they are more alkaline.

Prebiotics: Carbohydrates that selectively feed beneficial bacteria in the gut and thus support their growth and development. The most common prebiotics are inulin and FOS.

Probiotics: Microorganisms (bacteria in most cases) that promote life and health by protecting their host (you) against disease-causing organisms and supporting other life-enhancing functions. Perhaps the best-known probiotic is *Lactobacillus acidophilus*.

Protease: An enzyme that can break a protein into its components—peptides.

Proteolysis: The breakdown of proteins to form simpler, smaller substances.

Subspecies: A subdivision of a species.

Synbiotic: A supplement or food that contains both probiotics and prebiotics.

Resources

Do It Yourself Probiotics

Body Ecology.com
218 Laredo Drive
Decatur, GA 30030
800-511-2660

Information and starter kits for making your own fermented vegetables

Leeners
(Suppliers of kits and items to make fermented foods)
9293 Olde Eight Road
Northfield, OH 44067
800-543-3697
www.leeners.com

Bentley, Nancy Lee. *Fermented Foods for Health: Making and Enjoying Naturally Fermented Foods for Better Digestion and Overall Health.* Beverly, MA: Fair Winds, 2008.

Katz, Sandor. *Wild Fermentation: The Flavor, Nutrition and Craft of Live-Culture Foods.* White River Junction, VT: Chelsea Green Publishing, 2003.

Kaufmann, K. and Annelies Schoneck. *Making Sauerkraut and Pickled Vegetables at Home: Creative Recipes for Lactic Fermented Food to Improve Your Health.* British Columbia, Canada: Alive Books, 2002.

Probiotic and Synbiotic Foods

(NOTE: Information about CFUs and other product claims given below have been gathered from data supplied by the food manufacturers on their labels and/or Web sites. You should contact manufacturers individually if you have any questions about their products. Because probiotic and synbiotic foods is a rapidly growing area, you should be seeing many new products on the market.)

Brown Cow Farm
3810 Delta Fair Blvd
Antioch, CA 94509
888-429-5459
www.browncowfarm.com

Makers of yogurt that contains *S. thermophilus, L. bulgaricus, L. acidophilus,* and *B. bifidus*

Dannon
PO Box 90296
Allentown, PA 18109-0296
877-326-6668

Makers of various yogurt/probiotic products, including Activia™, a probiotic yogurt that contains a unique strain of bacteria (*Bifidus regularis*), and DanActive™, a probiotic beverage that contains more than 10 billion CFUs of *Lactobacillus casei* per serving.

Helios Nutrition, Ltd.
214 Main Street
Sauk Centre, MN 56378
888-343-5467
www.heliosnutrition.com

Makers of synbiotic kefir in five flavors.

Horizon Organic Dairy
PO Box 17577
Boulder, CO 80308-7577

Yogurt products contain *L. acidophilus, L. bulgaricus, L. casei, B. bifidus,* and *S. thermophilus;* their cottage cheese and sour cream contain *L. acidophilus* and *B. bifidus.*

Lifeway Foods
6431 West Oakton Avenue
Morton Grove, IL 60053
847-967-1010
info@lifeway.net

Makes kefir, some especially for children, plus kefir starter. Their kefir contains *Lactobacillus lactis, L. rhamnosus, L. plantarum, L. casei, L. acidophilus, Streptococcus diacetylactis, Saccharomyces florentinus, Leuconostoc cremoris, Bifidobacterium longum, B. breve,* as well as immunoglobulins isolated from cow colostrum, which provides immunity against intestinal pathogens. According to the company's Web site, the kefir contains 5 to 10 billion CFUs per serving.

Stonyfield Farms
Ten Burton Drive
Londonderry, NH 03053
1-800-776-2697

Makes synbiotic yogurt that contains six species of bacteria (*Streptococcus thermophilus, Lactobacillus bulgaricus, L. casei, L. acidophilus, L. reuteri,* and *Bifidobacterium* species), as well as the prebiotic inulin.

Supplement Sources

Arise and Shine Herbal Products
PO Box 400
Medford, OR 97501
800-688-2444
www.ariseandshine.com

American Biologics
1180 Walnut Avenue
Chula Vista, CA 91911
800-227-4458
www.americanbiologics.com

Provides probiotic and enzyme supplements.

Dr. Shahani's Probiotics
Nebraska Cultures, Inc.
1911 Trenton Court
Walnut Creek, CA 94596
877-377-4242
www.drshahani.com

Has several probiotic formulas.

Enzymes, Inc.
8500 NW River Park Dr., #227
Parkville, MO 64152
800-637-7893

Provides a line of enzyme nutritional supplements (Genuine N*Zimes) developed by Dr. Edward Howell, a world-known expert on enzyme research.

Herbal Remedies USA
225 N. Wolcott
Casper, WY 82601
information@herbalremedies.com
www.herbalremedies.com

A source of sodium chlorite.

Natural Wellness Centers of America, Inc.
2121 W. Crescent Avenue, Suite C
Anaheim, CA 92801
888-207-3480
www.naturalwellness.com

Offers probiotic, enzyme, and MSM supplements, as well as sodium chlorite liquid.

Oxygen America, Inc.
19640 West Dixie Hwy
Miami, FL 33180
305-933-4219
www.oxygenamerica.com

Ultra-Pet Products
2121 W. Crescent Ave. Suite C
Anaheim, CA 92801
888-207-3480
www.total-zymes.com

Offers probiotic and enzyme supplements for dogs, cats, horses, and small animals.

Universal Herbs, Inc./Source Naturals
33453 Western Avenue
Union City, CA 94587
510-324-2900

Source of sodium chlorite (Oxy Response).

Selected Readings

Alvarez-Olmos, M. I. and R. A. Oberhelman. Probiotic agents and infectious diseases: a modern perspective on a traditional therapy. *Clinical Infectious Diseases.* 2001; 32(11):1567–76.

Brudnak, Mark A. *The Probiotics Solution: Nature's Best-Kept Secret for Radiant Health.* St. Paul, MN: Dragon Door, 2005.

Cabana, M. D., A. L. Shane, C. Chao, et al. Probiotics in primary care pediatrics. *Clinical Pediatrics.* 2006; 45(5):405–10.

Dash, S. K. *The Consumer's Guide to Probiotics: The Complete Source Book.* Topanga, CA: Freedom Press, 2005.

Doron, S. and S. L. Gorbach. Probiotics: their role in the treatment and prevention of disease. *Expert Review of Anti-Infective Therapy.* 2006; 4(2):261–75.

Elmer, Gary W. *The Power of Probiotics: Improving Your Health with Beneficial Microbes.* Binghamton, NY: Haworth Press, 2007.

Ezendam, J. and H. van Loveren. Probiotics: immunomodulation and evaluation of safety and efficacy. *Nutrition Reviews.* 2006; 64(1):1–14.

Hammerman, C., A. Bin-Nun, M. Kaplan. Safety of probiotics: comparison of two popular strains. *BMJ.* 2006; 333(7576):1006–1008.

Huebner, E. S. and C. M. Surawicz. Probiotics in the prevention and treatment of gastrointestinal infections. *Gastroenterology Clinics of North America.* 2006; 35(2):355–365.

Huffnagle, Gary B. and Sarah Wernick. *The Probiotic Revolution: The Definitive Guide to Safe, Natural Health Solutions with Probiotic and Prebiotic Foods and Supplements.* New York: Bantam, 2007.

Karpa, Kelly D. *Bacteria for Breakfast: Probiotics for Good Health.* Victoria, Canada: Trafford Publishing, 2006.

Reid, G. and J. A. Hammond. Probiotics: some evidence of their effectiveness. *Canadian Family Physician.* 2005; 51:1487–93.

Salminen, S. J., M. Gueimonde and E. Isolauri. Probiotics that modify disease risk. *Journal of Nutrition.* 2005; 135(5):1294–1298.

Shahani, K. M. *Cultivate Health From Within: Dr. Shahani's Guide to Probiotics.* Danbury, CT: Vital Health Publishing, 2005.

Trenev, Natasha. *Probiotics: Nature's Internal Healers.* New York: Avery, 1998.

Index

Index

Index

DATE DUE

Demco, Inc. 38-293